AF248815

Ethical Issues in
Epidemiologic Research

Series in Psychosocial Epidemiology
Volume 7

ANDREW E. SLABY, M.D., Ph.D., M.P.H.
General Editor

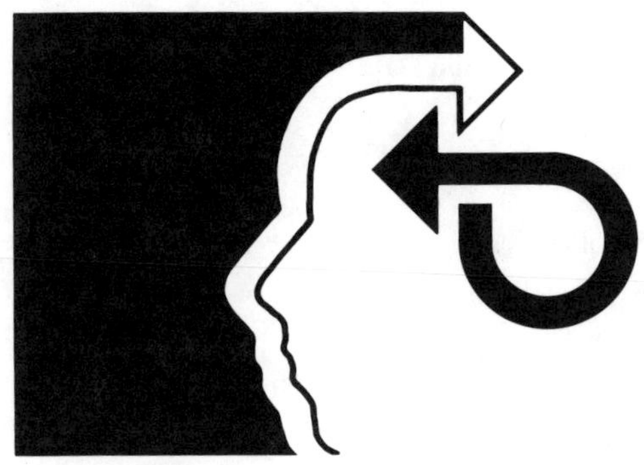

SERIES IN
PSYCHOSOCIAL
EPIDEMIOLOGY

VOLUME 7

ETHICAL ISSUES IN EPIDEMIOLOGIC RESEARCH

EDITED BY

Laurence Tancredi

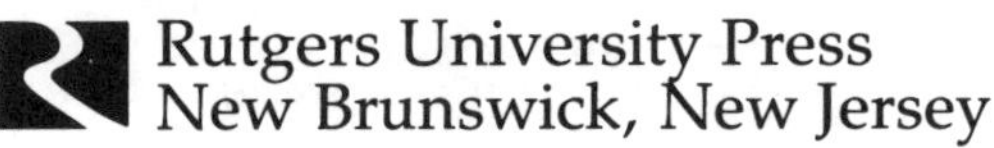Rutgers University Press
New Brunswick, New Jersey

Library of Congress Cataloging-in-Publication Data
Main entry under title:

Ethical issues in epidemiologic research.

   (Series in psychosocial epidemiology; v. 7)
   Includes bibliographies.
   1. Psychiatric epidemiology—Research—Moral and
ethical aspects. 2. Psychotherapy—Evaluation—
Research—Moral and ethical aspects. I. Tancredi,
Laurence R. II. Series. [DNLM: 1. Epidemiologic
Methods. 2. Ethics, Medical. 3. Health Policy—
United States. 4. Mental Disorders—occurrence—
United States. 5. Psychiatry—standards—United
States. 6. Research—standards—United States.
w1 PS79E v.7/WM 62 E843]
RC455.2.E64E84   1986   174'.2   85–27941
ISBN 0–8135–1156–9
ISBN 0–8135–1157–7 (pbk.)

Contents

Introduction to Studies in Psychosocial Epidemiology

Rising costs of mental health care and interest in the development of national health insurance that should include some mental health services have heightened concern both for ways by which health planners may evaluate the extent of behavioral problems and for means by which the efficacy of various treatment modalities may be assessed. Questions of paramount importance include: If there exist two or more ways of treating an illness, which is most effective? If two therapeutic modalities are equally effective, which is more efficient? If equally efficient, which is less costly? Comparable questions regarding the prevalence and incidence rates of specific psychiatric illness in communities are being raised by those delegated the task of making policy recommendations for programs of primary prevention and treatment. What is the natural history of an untreated behavioral problem and how is the problem affected by normal growth and development? What does knowledge of the natural history of a disorder of mood, thought, and behavior tell us about its etiology, and how may such knowledge lead to methods of prevention? If an illness is not preventable by currently available knowledge, what interventions may be made in its natural history to arrest and possibly reverse its course? Mental health is now big business; failure to look at specific population needs when planning programs and to include ways of evaluating cost-efficiency-effectiveness results in considerable psychological and economic cost to millions of patients and their families, as well as to taxpayers in general.

Epidemiology is a body of knowledge and technical skills that may be put to use in answering some of the questions facing health planners today. Traditionally, epidemiology has been seen as the study of disease patterns in populations. Epidemiologists have been useful in providing data that have led to effective programs of prevention of a number of infectious diseases including malaria, smallpox, and poliomyelitis. Epidemiology has, however, played a minor role in psychiatric research until relatively recently. Epidemiological studies in mental health tended to be descriptive and to focus on the prevalence and incidence rates of symptoms in broad categories of illness, such as "neuroses" or "psychoses." Some infectious- and chronic-disease epidemiologists, in fact, question whether epidemiology can be used to tackle psychiatric problems. The Society for Epidemiologic Research does not have a section on psychosocial epidemiology, and publication of papers in social and psychiatric epidemiology in its journal is infrequent. Principal organs of dispersion of knowledge in psychosocial epidemiology have been *Psychological Medicine* and the *Archives of General Psychiatry*. The former journal, published quarterly, has on its editorial board members sophisticated in epidemiology and probably publishes the greatest number of articles in this area. It, however, is a British journal with limited readership in the United States. On the other hand, the *Archives of General Psychiatry*, a publication of the American Medical Association, is fairly widely read in the United States. It publishes a number of high quality papers in epidemiology but has a broad mandate and, therefore, is limited in its ability to publish more.

The *Series in Psychosocial Epidemiology*, of which this is the seventh volume, is to serve several important functions for epidemiology, psychiatry, and related areas in public health. Its objectives include:

1. Providing a forum for discussion of research strategies in the evaluation of mental health problems in the community and for assessing the effectiveness of psychiatric treatment interventions,
2. Serving as a teaching tool for students in medical schools and schools of public health, hospital administration, social work, and nursing, as well as for students in departments of psychology, sociology, and especially epidemiology,
3. Keeping prospective researchers alert to problems needing investigation in the area of psychosocial epidemiology,
4. Serving as a vehicle to bring together research in the area of psychosocial epidemiology,

5. Providing a means of continuing education for epidemiologists working in the field,
6. Providing a means for discussion of how the results of epidemiological and related behavioral research might be
   brought to bear on the development of state and federal
   health policy decisions.

To achieve these ends, each volume has a single theme of particular interest to investigators in the field of psychosocial epidemiology, themes such as the study of children, the study of stressful life events, and needs assessment. Each volume in the series has a guest editor, with an established reputation in the field who has selected and edited contributions and written the introductory article. In general, in the lead article the guest editor (1) discusses methodological considerations for research in a given area (i.e., experimental design, sampling, instruments used, analysis of data, economic considerations, and ethical decisions in planning studies), (2) critically reviews existing studies, (3) presents information on the current state of the field, and (4) suggests directions for further research. Most volumes also provide an Afterword written by a representative of the World Health Organization (WHO) and an Introduction written by the series editor. The WHO representative, chosen by Dr. Norman Sartorius, Director of the Division of Mental Health, focuses on what is being done internationally in the topic area discussed; what should be done cooperatively and independently to advance the field; what WHO feels are research priorities in the field; and what particular methodological problems in research in the given area exist in pretechnological and third-world nations. I will direct the Foreword to the present state of epidemiological research in the area, the directions the Center for Epidemiologic Studies at the National Institute of Mental Health would like to see research take, and the relationship of research in the field to the formulation of health policy.

Following the present volume *Ethical Issues in Epidemiologic Research*, the series will include volumes on needs assessment, genetics, aging, and the methodology of natural experiments. Earlier volumes in the series focused on studies of children, stressful life events, help-seeking behavior, alcohol use studies, drug abuse studies, and community surveys. Barbara Dohrenwend, Bruce P. Dohrenwend, Felton Earls, Stanislav V. Kasl, David Mechanic, Jerome Myers, Lee N. Robins, Catherine E. Ross, Marc Schuckit, Laurence R. Tancredi, Ming T. Tsuang, George Warheit, and Myrna M. Weissman are the current guest editors.

The mandate of this series is challenging and the task great. However, with the help of the guest editors and other contributors the series can provide researchers, students, and health policy makers much of what they need to know about research in psychosocial epidemiology in order to plan future research and to design effective and consumer-responsive health policy and preventive psychiatric care programs.

A.E.S.

Foreword

Commitment to research is a *value* and an important one in efforts to advance the frontiers of understanding the etiology, treatment, and prevention of mental illness. Equally important, however, are the values placed on human rights to privacy, to informed consent, to treatment when ill, and to refuse treatment. Researchers in psychosocial epidemiology, as in other areas of research, endeavor to weigh the risks and benefits to the individual and to society of various research designs. Epidemiological research entails understanding the course of an untreated illness in order to evaluate the efficacy of preventive or therapeutic interventions.

To reveal the history of an untreated illness, treatment must be withheld. This raises serious ethical questions when some modality, albeit limited, may alleviate the distress caused by illness to patient or family. These are new problems for psychiatric researchers. Until a few decades ago, neither diagnostic techniques nor quantification of therapeutic endeavors were sufficiently elaborated to provide the data needed to evaluate the efficacy of modern therapeutic interventions. For instance, the evaluation of the roles of psychotherapy, sociotherapy, psychopharmacotherapy, and electroshock in the management of depression entails reliable and valid techniques for identifying patients with the type of depression to be studied, knowledge of the duration of an untreated depressive episode and quantification of observed psychological, physical, and social changes. Drugs may affect psychological and biological changes, such as felt depression, sleep disturbances, and changes in appetite and libido, but not social adjustment. The last may be affected more by sociotherapy and psychotherapy, but only after the neurovegetative symptoms and signs (sleep and appetite disturbances) of depression have been alleviated by medication. There is an ethical responsibility to both patients and care-givers to accurately define the illness and the treatment interventions in order to give interventions a fair trial. The success of some interventions like electroshock, as Tancredi tells us, may be impressive in the short run, but less effective than psychopharmacotherapy for long-term relief.

An understanding of the natural history of an illness may be obtained both retrospectively and prospectively. Retrospective studies are usually weaker in design but are necessary because of time and economic constraints. Chart review is one retrospective approach, but resulting information suffers from the recording biases of clinicians and the limited ability of patients and relatives to recall past life circumstances. Access to records presents problems in confidentiality, informed consent, and privacy. The alternative and generally favored approach, prospective studies with a follow-up design, may present not only problems of confidentiality but special problems of following high-risk individuals.

The evaluation of the efficacy of a clinical intervention raises yet another set of unique ethical considerations, ranging from the statistical need for randomization of clinical trials and large samples to the need for a long enough intervention to allow a just assessment of its efficacy. Contributors to this volume explore various problems of particular interest to investigators in psychosocial epidemiology.

In chapter 1, Laurence R. Tancredi discusses how the use of epidemiological methods for assessing medical practices has increased in importance with the expansion of therapeutic interventions, from medications to highly expensive procedures and assist devices, and the increasing accountability to society for cost-efficiency-effectiveness through third party reimbursement agencies (in particular, Medicare and Medicaid) in the payment of health services. Tancredi underscores the fact that, while the natural history of a disease must be understood to evaluate the efficiency and effectiveness of medical interventions with psychotropic drugs in the 1950s, there has been little opportunity to do so. Prior to the fifties, depression and schizoprenia were used as catchall phrases for a number of diseases. Only with the development of modern epidemiological techniques, such as those discussed by Weissman and Myers in volume 4 of this series, on Community Surveys, have we been able to isolate the parameters of an illness that may selectively respond to therapeutic interventions. For example, the neurovegetative signs of unipolar affective illness respond to antidepressant drugs. Psychotherapy and sociotherapy act to enhance social adjustment, while doing little for the neurovegetative symptoms, but only after the antidepressant medication has taken effect. Psychiatric research, particularly that involving drugs and psychotherapy, as Tancredi points out, has become very value laden. Psychotherapy no doubt plays an important role in the management of a number of psychiatric illnesses, but proof of its effectiveness requires studies designed to define the therapy in terms of duration, frequency, provider, and type. Moreover, the populations served must be appropriately characterized, and the most effective time to introduce treatment must be detailed. Tancredi cautions against early termination of a study before an intervention may have been given sufficient time to manifest meaningful results simply because the traditional treatment used as a control appeared to be far more effective in the early phases of an illness. This can be illustrated by comparative studies of the efficacy of tricyclic and tetracyclic antidepressants and monoamine oxidase inhibitors versus electroshock in the treatment of severe depression. The therapeutic impact of the medication is very time dependent, not maximized until three to six weeks of therapeutic doses. A prematurely ended investigation would lead to the erroneous conclusion that electroshock is the universally superior mode of treatment.

Drugs do have serious side effects. The most dramatic are the cardiovascular side effects of antidepressants and the long-term neurological changes (e.g., tardive dyskinesia) seen in some patients on antipsychotic medication. Yet, controlled clinical trials now show that more and more illnesses, previously considered predominantly psychological in origin, respond to drug interventions. Phobias and obsessive-compulsive neuroses once thought to respond only to behavioral interventions have been relieved by such drugs as imipramine, propranolol, and monoamine oxidase inhibitors. To patients this means a welcome reduction of both human suffering and the costs of long-term treatments often of uncertain efficacy.

Tancredi discusses in some detail three major ethical issues bearing on epidemiological research: informed consent, confidentiality, and the right to refuse treatment. A unique problem in psychosocial epidemiology is that often the most relevant populations for study (e.g., children and the mentally ill) cannot provide truly informed consent themselves. Assuming that scientifically accurate studies have been performed and information gleaned regarding risk, benefits, and alternatives to treatment, it is important that patients be placed in the best position to give informed consent. In the discussion of confidentiality of information, Tancredi reviews the implications of the *Tarasoff* case, where the courts imposed an obligation on therapists and investigators to warn patients who may risk potential physical harm. His discussion of the right to refuse treatment focuses on the importance of the information made available to patients so that, in accordance with the rules promulgated by the national Institutes of Health, they can withdraw from the experiment at any point and refuse the treatment being offered.

Walter Reich, in chapter 2, discusses the ethical need for reliable and valid diagnostic schema in psychiatry and the potential of diagnostic schema for societal abuse. Diagnosis is needed to dictate treatment and for empirical psychiatric research, but it has its limits. The simplest source of misdiagnosis lies in the vulnerability of the diagnostic process to inconsistency and change, a reliance on subjective criteria, and bias. Because physicians as a group feel that a Type 2 error (accepting a false hypothesis) is less dangerous than a Type 1 error (rejecting a true hypothesis), the process is biased toward the diagnosis of health rather than illness. Reich also illustrates some abuses of the diagnostic process, including the use of a diagnosis for explanation, mitigation, and exculpation; for reassurance; for the humane transformation of social deviance into medical illness; for exclusion and dehumanization; to support self-confirming hypotheses; and for discreditation and punishment. He uses the experience of psychiatry in the Soviet Union to demonstrate how an official diagnostic system can shape psychiatric vision and ensnare individuals, who elsewhere would be considered mentally well, in a broad net that irrevocably defines them as psychiatrically ill. The Soviet experience, Reich contends, is important in that it exemplifies in a pure and extreme form a trend only now developing in other countries, including the United States. It illustrates with poignant clarity how a system that appears to have only a scientific basis and professional goals can simply, by virtue of its own nature as a systematic technology, result in significant abuse. Soviet patients may be diagnosed as schizophrenic even if they exhibit no signs of an illness, and once the diagnosis is given, even if it is further subtyped as mild, it continues to be employed with the tacit assumption that the individual has a life-long genetically based condition.

Deinstitutionalization is a public policy based on several empirically validated findings. Patients in long-term hospitals, even private and richly staffed facilities, undergo a social deterioration variously labeled as deculturation, institutionalism, or the social breakdown syndrome. These changes are felt to be an outcome of confinement in total institutions with a hierarchical organization of behavioral accountability, rather than a manifestation of the alterations in social functioning that are part and parcel of such illnesses as chronic schizophrenia. These findings, coupled with a real desire to provide more humane and less costly alternatives to traditional psychiatric care, led well-meaning health policy makers to adopt deinstitutionalization. Unfortunately, the move toward community care took place before adequate community facilities and services to receive patients were available and without prior consideration that patients who have had years of institutionalized care may be less able to adjust to community life than more recently ill patients who have never been hospitalized for lengthy periods.

Michels and Eth, in chapter 3, examine some of the ethical issues raised by the shift in mental health policy inherent in the community mental health movement and the deinstitutionalization of psychiatric patients. They focus attention on the unique ethical problems that emerge in community level interventions. Patients, without prior consent by them or the community, have been required to leave institutions that were "home." Often, their relatives were without resources to receive them and were suffering from psychiatric illness themselves; also the patients were frequently financially and physically constrained by the infirmities of old age. On the positive side, one would expect to see less social deterioration of patients and a beneficial change in public attitudes toward mental illness if a policy of community-based care is successfully implemented. Whether the cost of care for attendant health and social services will be reduced is still questionable.

Lee N. Robins, in chapter 4, addresses the consequences of the recommendations of the Privacy Protection Study Commission for longitudinal studies. While aggregate and anonymous records are useful to many kinds of social research, in longitudinal studies individually identifiable records must be available for sampling, locating subjects for interview, tracing additional records relating to the subjects, verifying interview data, and obtaining data for their own sake. Those who disapprove allowing researchers access to identifiable records argue that the same populations can be longitudinally studied without individual links. Evidence suggests, however, that this is not the case. Robins points out that turnover tables of alcohol abuse show that the level of problem drinking in the population is quite constant over time but that different people are involved at different times. What contributed to remission and to late onset will not be revealed if rates of alcoholism are available only for the population as a whole. If epidemiological knowledge is to be advanced, researchers must have access to records and not merely to abstracts made by disinterested others. They must also have some idea in each case of the risks and benefits of disclosure of such information. There is a burden on researchers to provide an appropriate rationale for such research to provide safeguards around confidentiality, and to destroy sensitive data when no longer needed.

The ethics of research on subjects at high risk of schizophrenia is the subject of chapter 5 by Natalie Abrams. Schizophrenia is not simply an inherited disease. Not everyone who possesses the suspected genotype becomes schizophrenic. Studies of monozygotic twins indicate that one may develop the disease while the other may not. This suggests that, while the development of schizophrenia may in part depend upon possession of the requisite genotype, environmental factors play a critical role. High-risk research aims at identifying both genetic and environmental factors.

Cross-sectional retrospective studies are fraught with errors in reporting. Parents may interpret rather than accurately report past experiences in an attempt to explain a child's present behavior. In such attempts to explain, some parents may also recall and place significance on past incidents that other parents would not remember. Parents are not always able to take a realistic view of their own behavior and consequently either exaggerate or fail to recognize their own personal mode of interaction, or simply recall situations incorrectly. Prospective follow-up studies of high-risk children over a number of years, using controls who do not have a history of mental illness in the family, provide a stronger research model for determining what factors contribute to the development of mental illness. In such situations, information about early life is more accurate and the temporal relationship between environmental factors and the development of psychiatric disorders more readily discernible. In addition, a more complete sample of the population can be achieved.

Ethical problems confronting researchers interested in following high-risk populations include issues of autonomy and consent, privacy, acceptable levels of risk, and the principle of liberty. Children need "proxy" consent. Research is not therapeutic and may lead to a self-fulfilling prophecy. A particularly serious issue is whether questioning normal children, especially those whose parents are schizophenic, could cause the children to become anxious and overly concerned about their future development and even their present psychological state. Abrams states that this risk is highlighted by the fact that many of the children are interviewed during their pre-adolescent and adolescent periods, when a normal child is frequently having self-doubts and going through emotional and physiological changes. At such a time, it may not be in the best interests of the children to have their psychological status probed by psychiatric personnel or for them to feel that they will be followed throughout the course of their development. Could such interviewing and questioning indirectly cause the behavior observed in studies of the concept of self-fulfilling prophecy?

Lindenthal and Thomas, chapter 6, review some of the dilemmas and sources of difficulty in handling confidentiality in clinical settings. They discuss attitudes and values regarding this issue, as well as official positions taken by professional organizations in psychiatry and psychology. Tancredi and Weisstub, chapter 7, examine the effect of ideologies on the design, the implementation, and, ultimately, the interpretation of epidemiological studies in forensic psychiatry. As data from such research are increasingly used by courts in decisions affecting the mental health care system, the distorting impact of ideological influences introduces major ethical problems. In the final chapter, Alexander Brooks discusses the constitutional right to refuse antipsychotic medication. Antipsychotic drugs are unequivocally effective in the management of acute symptoms of psychosis but also have untoward effects, including tardive dyskinesia, a potentially irreversible neurological process. Changes in legislation regarding a patient's rights to receive appropriate treatment and to refuse undesired treatment have considerable consequences for those interested in clinical epidemiological research.

All human research has social and individual implications. All researchers have social and scientific responsibilities. An epidemiological researcher must balance the risks and benefits of the research to society and to individual subjects. Research can never be reviewed in a vacuum. We are where we are today in preventive medicine and psychiatry because those before us weighed such risks and performed such research. We owe to those who follow us a legacy of responsibly acquired scientific knowledge like that our predecessors left us.

A.E.S.

Ethical Issues in
Epidemiologic Research

Chapter 1

The New Technology of Psychiatry: Ethics, Epidemiology, and Technology Assessment

LAURENCE TANCREDI

Since the development of the artificial kidney and organ transplantation during the 1960s, the assessment of new medical technologies—diagnostic and treatment techniques as well as innovative designs in the delivery of health services—has become critically important in the health care field. These technologies have not only enhanced the quality of diagnosis and treatment of diseases but have become a major factor, primarily through Medicare and Medicaid, in the ever-increasing involvement of society in the payment for health services. In psychiatry, such technologies were previously limited to physical therapies, such as psychosurgery, insulin shock, and electroshock, and verbal therapies such as psychoanalysis. Over the past thirty years the technologies in psychiatry have become principally biological in nature and now include a wide range of powerful psychotropic medications—antidepressants and antipsychotics.

The most important tools for the assessment of medical practices are epidemiological methods. These methods have long been applied to medical events in order to understand the natural history of disease, but their role in evaluating the efficacy of medical services is relatively new. To achieve a description of the net benefits and risks of therapeutic interventions, it is essential that information be collected about the natural history of various diseases to serve as a baseline against which the advantages of proposed treatments can be compared (Frazer & Hiatt, 1978).

With regard to the historical role of epidemiology, that is, for

1

understanding the natural history of various diseases, prominent deficiencies in knowledge remain, especially of the chronic illnesses and, most particularly, psychiatric diseases. Since the advent of psychotropic medications in the fifties and sixties, there has been little opportunity to observe both individually and epidemiologically the trajectory of many mental illnesses. Furthermore, as emphasized by Frazer & Hiatt (1978), we have little understanding of the natural history of medical diseases. To illustrate this assertion, they allude to the fact that it was not known until the mid-1950s that more than 70 percent of individuals afflicted with untreated syphilis died without any evidence of the disease. Eighty-five percent of those with untreated syphilis lived essentially normal lives. In psychiatry, the natural history of diseases such as schizophrenia and the affective disorders was established at a time when psychiatric sciences were not sophisticated about epidemiological techniques, but relied on clinical experiences with individual patients. In addition, terms like schizophrenia until recently were unitary concepts that became catchall phrases for a wide range of psychotic processes that have been subsequently subjected to more careful differentiation.

Our knowledge about the efficacy and effectiveness of various treatments has been muddied by conceptual limitations. Most particularly, the point of contrast for examining the effectiveness of new techniques has relied upon an insufficiently studied and described history of the untreated diseases. In addition to this limitation are those problems introduced by the fact that outcomes of treatment are highly value laden. For example, the measurement of whether a particular drug is effective in the treatment of manic depressive illness may be skewed by unconscious biases or the way in which patients have been selected. Many of these treatments have never been put to well-designed clinical trials large enough to be statistically significant. Even in general medicine, where randomized clinical trials and other designs for assessment have had a longer history of application than in psychiatry, several technological achievements in treatment became commonplace and accepted without being thoroughly assessed through well-designed clinical trials. One of the most conspicuous of such treatments was the use of coronary care units for uncomplicated myocardial infarctions. Mather and colleagues (Mather et al., 1971, 1976) in a study in England established that patients suffering from uncomplicated myocardial infarctions could be adequately cared for in their homes with a mortality rate that was certainly no greater than would be found in a hospital or coronary care unit. The use of radical mastectomies for cancer of the breast is another treatment that has come under scrutiny. This operation is still widely practiced in this country, but evidence indicates that it may be no more effective than simple operative procedures (Bunker, et al., 1977). Results of a randomized clinical trial recently conducted to evaluate the effectiveness of coronary artery by-pass graft surgical procedures suggest that this technique may be medically applicable only to a very small or well-circumscribed group of patients (Murphy et al., 1977). Many patients now receiving this procedure are unlikely to benefit significantly in terms of myocardial functioning.

Historically, it has been very difficult, if not impossible, to evaluate the effectiveness of the wide range of verbal therapies used in psychiatric practice. Attempts have been made to assess outcomes for psychotherapy, but these measurements are even more value-laden than in other areas of medical practice (Cochran, 1972). The endpoints to be achieved in psychotherapy have by no means been universally agreed upon. One need only examine some of the writings of leaders of the various schools of psychiatry to discover the broad range of meanings ascribed to "mental health" and "normality" (Tancredi & Slaby, 1977). For some practitioners, patients benefit from treatment to the extent that they are able to "self-actualize" and thus gain greater power over their own destiny. Others set a more limited goal, such as modifying certain behaviors that create mental and emotional problems for the patient. And for others yet more pragmatically oriented, the aim may simply be finding ways to mitigate the anxiety or other symptoms that result from characterological or neurotic processes. In any case, a survey of the many psychiatrists and psychotherapists providing care for the mentally and emotionally ill would result in a diverse description of the expected benefits from treatment.

From another perspective, however, psychiatry has in many respects become more akin to other areas of medical practice. For some time physically active procedures such as electroshock therapy, insulin therapy, and certain forms of psychosurgery have been used on patients. But in recent years the fastest grow-

ing area of psychiatric intervention is the use of medications—
mood-stabilizing and anti-anxiety agents and neuroleptic drugs
for serious as well as minimally symptomatic psychiatric illness.
These drugs are not without costs and potential risks to the patient as well as the health care system in general. Because of this
ever-expanding armamentarium of psychiatric therapeutics,
there is a critical need for epidemiological evaluation of the underlying diseases being treated and of the treatments currently
in use. Such evaluation must take into account the effectiveness
of these medications as contrasted with absence of treatment
or more traditional treatments such as psychotherapy, milieu
therapy, and other methods. In addition, determining efficacy
includes examining how well the technology works in various
health care settings, e.g., university medical centers, small community hospitals, and private practice and when administered
by other mental health professionals.

This discussion is concerned with some of the underlying ethical and social issues associated with the application of epidemiological techniques in psychiatry. Primary emphasis is placed on
the ethical issues surrounding the use of random clinical trials
for the expansion of available information regarding certain diseases and treatment processes. The first part of this discussion
focuses on what is known about the nature of various studies
that deal with the effectiveness and efficacy of treatments. Since
most of the work in this area has been done in general medical
services, it will be necessary to rely heavily on that body of literature to illustrate ethical issues that also pertain to psychiatry.
The second section deals with problems of informed consent.
Assuming that scientifically accurate studies are conducted, and
information has been gleaned regarding treatment benefits,
risks, and alternatives, it is important to assure that patients are
placed in the best position to give informed consent. Various
conceptual difficulties arise. These are discussed with particular emphasis on problems that prevent patients from having
sufficient power to make their own medical decisions. Included
in this discussion are an examination of the use of technology
assessment for determining the more effective use of psychiatric
manpower, specifically the use of criteria mapping or algorithms
in psychiatric practice, and informed consent requirements in
human experimentation.

The third part of the discussion is a brief review of two important issues that affect epidemiological research—confidentiality of information and the right to refuse treatment. With respect to confidentiality the emphasis is on current requirements, particularly as they may influence the conducting of important epidemiological studies. This includes a discussion of new developments, such as the *Tarasoff* case, that impose a duty on therapists and investigators to warn others of possible injury from dangerous patients. Discussion of the right to refuse treatment focuses on the importance of the information made available to patients so that, in accordance with rules promulgated by the National Institutes of Health, they can, if they wish, withdraw at any point in an experiment or refuse offered treatment.

Randomized Clinical Trials and Technology Assessment

One of the most important obligations of the medical profession is to test its assumptions about the diagnosis and treatment of disease. This has been done chiefly through individual case studies, but such studies have proved to be limited in that they do not reflect the full range of patient variability in diagnosis and response to treatment. Factors like the physician's degree of enthusiasm, the placebo effect, and differences in the virulence of the disease, which make it exceedingly difficult to generalize about treatment efficacy on the basis of a small number of cases, are not picked up in individual case studies (Tukey, 1977). Hence, broad-scale clinical trials are essential to protect the full interests of patients in the health care system. The profession has the responsibility to adequately test its assumptions with the most accurate and precise methods available and to assure that the information resulting from studies is made available to consumers of health services.

One of the benefits achieved by technology assessment is that, in addition to expanding available information regarding a new technology under consideration, comparative studies with traditional therapies as controls yield assessments of existing diagnostic procedures and treatment used in current medical practice. For example, when a drug is introduced for the treatment of psychotic depression, proper technology assessment involves examining the extent to which the drug controls symptoms and also, taking into consideration the full range of benefits and risks, the extent to which it is competitive with available alternatives. Having subjected new technological developments to stringent and precise testing, the profession then has a responsibility to incorporate into practice those that on balance have advantages over existing procedures.

Randomized clinical trials, especially double-blind cross-over types, are superior to other uncontrolled experiments in protecting the interests of patients because, if properly conducted, they give the most unbiased information about the effectiveness of therapies. They are likely to be most helpful in dealing with new therapies whose medical value is uncertain or with existing therapies whose relative benefits are in dispute (Byar et al., 1976).

Randomized clinical trials have three advantages: First, they eliminate as much as possible a conscious or unconscious bias in the selection of patients for a particular form of treatment since the patients are arbitrarily placed in specific treatment protocols.

Second, randomization tends to make treatment groups more comparable. Third, along the same lines, randomization enhances the validity of the statistical test of significance applied to the assessment of compared treatments. Though the groups to be compared are never perfectly balanced to eliminate differences, randomization allows the descriptions of a probability distribution for differences and outcomes where equally effective treatments are used.

Other Research Methods

Some scholars disagree with the insistence on the merits of randomized clinical trials, claiming that quantitative comparative clinical trials can be achieved through other methods such as selection of literature controls, match controls, or controls from previous studies (Gahen & Freireich, 1974). They argue that such control studies have permitted assessment of the therapeutic efficacy of many anticarcinogenic agents. Furthermore, they say that randomization is perhaps most beneficial when a pilot study has indicated major differences in response rates for a particular treatment, and it is desired to establish the treatment's effectiveness more definitively. Along the same lines of argument, they claim that random clinical trials may be indicated if the new proposed therapy would be of benefit only if substantially better than existing therapies.

These authors claim particularly that some nonrandomized control studies can achieve the same ends as randomized studies when the intent is not to evaluate relative effectiveness but to show significant differences. The conceptual difficulty with this argument, however, is that it evades the high potential for bias in nonrandomized studies which rely on personal reports of therapeutic achievements. As we have already seen in Frazer & Hiatt (1978), the outcomes of many medical treatments in past studies seem to be highly value laden, yet the treatments are often adhered to as quality care, even in the face of contradictory evidence that alternative or perhaps less risky procedures would be equally, if not more, effective. In contrast, a properly conducted randomized clinical trial promotes scientific objectivity and is more likely to protect the interests of patients in obtaining the highest quality treatment available.

Accuracy in Research

In addition to the ethical issues involved in the proper design of scientifically valid clinical studies, it is important to follow strict statistical rules regarding both the sample size and duration of studies so that they may be carried to a stage where they are likely to yield good results. An equally perplexing concern is that studies be conducted at an appropriate time in the development of and dissemination of information about the new therapy to be tested. Freiman et al. (1978) examined 71 "negative" randomized clinical trials to try to determine what was responsible for the negative results. They learned that 67 of these studies had a 10-percent chance of missing as much as 25-percent improvement resulting from therapy. In addition, they estimated that at least 50 of the studies may well have missed a 50-percent improvement. One interesting observation was that a large percentage of the 71 negative randomized clinical trials involved too small a sample size to give meaningful data. Also, some of the studies were terminated well before they could achieve significant results simply because early indications implied that the traditional treatment used as a control was far more effective than the new treatment.

An example of how such premature termination might happen in psychiatric therapy is the comparison of a tricyclic antidepressant with electroshock in the treatment of severe depression. If the investigation ends before the medication is likely to have its most effective therapeutic impact, which is very time dependent, one would be led to the conclusion that electroshock treatment is far superior. However, studies have shown that antidepressant medication can be very effective but must be administered at a therapeutic dosage for six weeks to three months before conclusions can be drawn about its therapeutic efficacy. Terminating the study earlier would distort the statistical results. It is conceivable that many psychiatric therapies may have been and will be discarded as ineffective because of improperly designed or insufficiently prolonged studies.

The timing of assessments can be crucial. Treatments in their very early stages must not be subjected to definitive randomized clinical trials if there is a danger that the results might bias against the treatment before it has undergone the developments and changes almost inevitable for any new technology. Boncheck (1979) demonstrated the possible pitfalls of subjecting technologies too early to intensive randomized clinical trials. In a review of various important surgical procedures, he showed that randomized clinical trials conducted during the very early stages of new medical technologies may produce misleading negative results that do not reflect refinements developed during the course of the investigation. He demonstrated that reviewing mortality rates of various worthy but prematurely evaluated procedures may give the impression that these procedures are not effective. He showed that comparative evaluations in the early stages of some selective surgical operations indicated very high mortality rates which fell dramatically with later improvements in technique. His examples mostly involved cardiac surgery. He pointed out that during the late sixties, in the early stages of the development of coronary by-pass surgery, the mortality rate was nearly 12 percent in a very small group of patients. By the early and mid-seventies, the rate had dropped to 1.5 percent. Mitral commissurotomy, almost universally fatal during the early days of its application to the treatment of mitral stenosis, now also has a very low mortality rate. Boncheck's last example, mitral valve replacement, was first reported to have a mortality rate of 15 to 20 percent; this has decreased considerably in the past ten years.

In addition to the issues of sample size, length of study, and timing relevant to randomized clinical trials, the question arises as to which events should be counted to arrive at valid and useful data. In an article on the controversy in counting and attributing events in clinical trials, Sackett & Gent (1979) presented several illustrations of studies whose results made no sense when one examined how they counted certain events. In one example, a study of extracranial artery occlusion statistically compared the results of surgical and nonsurgical treatment of transient cerebral ischemic attacks in patients with bilateral carotid stenosis. Since the study restricted its analysis of comparative benefits to those patients "available for follow-up," the results showed, as might be expected, significantly less risk of recurrent transient ischemic attacks or strokes following the operation. However, the group "available for follow-up" included only patients discharged alive and free of sequelae following initial hospitalization, thus excluding some patients who died during the initial hospitalization or suffered additional strokes. When such individuals were included in the study, the results did not show overwhelming benefits of the operation for patients suffering from bilateral carotid stenosis.

From another perspective, of course, to count every event from the time the patients have been randomized may create equally skewed results. For example, the authors point to a study comparing the use of streptokinase and heparin for the treatment of acute myocardial infarction, whose results suggested that streptokinase significantly reduced mortality. However, a large number of patients who died after randomization but before receiving a test medication were all counted as part of the heparin group, even though none had received heparin. The resulting data give the impression that the patients treated with heparin for acute myocardial infarction had a significantly less optimistic outcome than patients treated with streptokinase. On closer scrutiny, of course, it is apparent that the many deaths incorrectly attributed to the heparin group tilted the scale against heparin.

Another complication may adversely affect the results of trials when insufficient attention is paid to possible variations in the medical responses of discrete groups of patients to specific treatments. Specifically, the authors pointed to the fact that including all hypertensive patients in a study of the effectiveness of a specific antihypertensive drug may distort the findings. It may be that the drug benefits only a small proportion of hypertensive patients. If the test involves all high blood pressure patients without discrimination, the specific drug may easily appear ineffective. For example, an antihypertensive drug may reduce the development of strokes and heart failure but have no influence on the development of coronary disease. Hence the drug may benefit some groups in a broad population of hypertensive patients but not others. The authors concluded that the resolution of this issue really rests in examining the underlying problems posed by the research if one is to avert distorting the evaluation of specific therapies. What is most important is to avoid the conclusion that a drug or agent is therapeutically effective when, in fact, it may be no better than a placebo, and, also, the conclusion that a therapy is not beneficial when, in fact, it has not been properly tested on specific discrete population groups for whom it may very well be a valuable treatment.

Sackett & Gent concluded that the determination of who should be included in a study depends on its objectives. For example, some studies are explanatory, attempting to demonstrate whether a given drug can bring about a specific outcome, such as preventing coronary occlusions, when administered under ideal circumstances. The objective here is to establish whether, if a trial is properly conducted, the medication does, in fact, produce a certain result. In psychiatry, one may want to know if a drug like lithium carbonate given under ideal circumstances will reduce cyclic mood disorders. If this is the objective, then it may be justifiable, according to Sackett & Gent, to limit patients to those most likely to comply with the prescribed medical regimen. On the other hand, a study may focus on assessing issues of therapeutic management. One such issue might be whether a therapy will work under clinical circumstances, taking into account all the good and bad consequences of such treatment conditions. This type of trial would justify accepting all individuals, even those known to comply poorly with medication regimens, in order to evaluate the overall usefulness of the treatment for a specific disease.

With these examples, Sackett & Gent effectively established

how important it is to be clear about the objectives of a research study so that only those individuals are included who will provide meaningful results, and events are counted at a stage that will yield valid conclusions. From the standpoint of ethics, anything short of precision in the execution of a study and the chosen scope of included subjects is inappropriate since the results would be of questionable scientific merit.

Evidence that many epidemiological studies have weak research designs was provided in an article by Fletcher & Fletcher (1979). These investigators examined over 600 randomly selected articles of original research published in *Lancet*, the *New England Journal of Medicine*, and the *Journal of the American Medical Association* between 1946 and 1976. They discovered that not only had weak research designs increased in frequency but that in 1976 the predominant research design was methodologically less accurate than randomized controlled trials. This discovery, based on three of the leading medical journals reporting clinical research in the medical care field, highlights the pervasiveness of poorly constructed studies and the inaccuracy of conclusions based on them.

Placebo Effect

One of the most controversial issues in the design of randomized clinical trials is the use of the placebo as a means of establishing that the treatment does more than just impact psychologically on patients. Some ethicists argue that the use of the placebo poses many ethical questions, most particularly those dealing with honesty and trust between the investigator and the patient (Bok, 1974; Simmons, 1978). They point to egregiously deceptive uses of the placebo in the care of patients or in human experimentation. One such study, conducted in the early seventies, involved a double-blind experiment with 76 women who entered a clinic for the purpose of preventing conception (Goldzieher, et al., 1971). The women were divided into two groups, one group receiving an oral contraceptive and a control group receiving a placebo. The control group was informed that their medication might not be completely effective in preventing conception and that, as a precaution, they should also use vaginal creams. They were not told that they were not receiving an oral contraceptive. The objective of the study was to determine whether patients receiving placebos would have the same undesirable side effects as those receiving a hormonal contraceptive agent, which would suggest that many of the undesirable effects may be psychologically induced. The results of this experiment demonstrated that psychological considerations do enter into the development of undesirable side effects from hormonal contraceptive agents but also included at least seven pregnancies among the control group.

The importance of addressing the placebo effect in randomized clinical trials cannot be underestimated, particularly when no alternative treatments are available that can be used for comparison in establishing the efficacy of a new technology. Critics of the use of the placebo claim that the patient participating in a research project should be informed that a placebo may be one of the alternative treatments. Of course, it might appear that telling patients they may be receiving a placebo would considerably affect the outcome of the experiment and obscure the influence of therapist enthusiasm and patient suggestibility. Some researchers argue that even patients aware of the possibility that they are receiving a placebo may still benefit from its administration (Park et al., 1967). One alternative to simply informing patients of the use of placebos is a modification of a proposal by Zelen (1979) that patients involved in randomized clinical trials be informed and allowed the alternative of consenting to the experimental treatment or being placed in a control group. The modification would be to so inform patients and then give them the opportunity, should they object to placebos, to enter a control group that will receive traditional therapy only. Analysis of the placebo effect is particularly important in psychiatric treatments, since the indicia of therapeutic efficacy rest on assessments of psychological states. Those assessing whether an antidepressant is effective in the treatment of serious depressive illness must consider not only the drug's impact on vegetative symptoms but the patient's own perception of well being. This perception can be strongly influenced by the relationship between patient and therapist and the degree of enthusiasm evidenced by the therapist regarding the medication in question.

In summary, the design and execution of research projects must deal with significant ethical and value issues. Since information obtained from such studies is critical to the interests of patients and consumers of health services, the studies must be precisely planned and properly conducted so that they provide meaningful data for evaluating the benefits and risks of various diagnostic and therapeutic modalities. The expansion of information through randomized clinical trials applies to traditional therapies as well as new technological developments. As knowledge increases, it will inevitably result in a reconceptualization of the goals of various treatments for psychiatric patients. Furthermore, properly conducted randomized clinical trials increase the amount of reliable information available to the patient in the therapeutic relationship, providing a stronger basis for truly informed consent.

Information Disclosure and Informed Consent

Many of the issues relevant to a physician-patient relationship with regard to informed consent also apply to epidemiological studies in psychiatry. The notion of informed consent was first introduced into American case law in the mid-fifties (*Salgo v. Leland Stanford, Jr., University Board of Trustees*, 1957). Since that time, nearly continuous attention has been given to the adequacy of this protective device for the patient in the therapeutic relationship. It has been argued by many that the doctrine of informed consent guards the individuality and autonomy of patients in the medical care system by affirming their prerogative to determine what is to be done with their physical and psychic integrity. Most importantly, it has been asserted that informed consent protects the individual's right to privacy, essentially the right to be left alone (Meisel, 1979). And finally, informed consent appears to be the cornerstone of the structure of patients' rights and power to gain control over what happens to them when they seek health care services.

From the viewpoint of human experimentation, there has been considerable expansion of the doctrine of informed consent, including requirements such as a full description of the proposed research, an examination of its intent and foreseeable benefits and risks, and a statement of available alternative procedures or treatments. Recent proposals go even farther and require that an institutional review board (IRB) review *all* research conducted on human subjects, not just projects supported by the federal health department. In addition, these proposed regulations require that the patient or subject of an experiment be informed by the institution or researcher as to what medical treatment and compensation would be made available, if any, should an injury occur. The patient should be told, according to this provision, whether the institution will pay for emergency care and compensation for functional loss and loss of wages or whether the patient will have to pay for such care in case of injury (Protection of Human Research Subjects, 1979).

With respect to research involving particularly vulnerable groups in the population, such as the mentally disabled, retarded, and children, proposals for even greater protection have been considered at various times (Protection of Human Subjects, 1978). One such proposal in the late seventies introduced two categories of risk that must be dealt with differently—"minimal risk" and "more than minimal risk" (Report and Recommendations of the National Commission for the Protection of Human Subjects of Biomedical and Behavioral Research, 1978). Two "levels of consent" were also proposed, based on the degree of risk and potential benefits of the therapy for the patient. One level refers to a capacity for "assent" that is essentially the ability to differentiate between "yes" and "no." The second level, referred to as "consent," is a greater degree of awareness in which the individual is competent enough to understand provided information and able to give a reasoned response. To provide greater protection around both "assent" and "consent," related largely to potential patient benefits and degree of risk, the proposal also allows for patient advocates, often referred to as "consent advocates." In addition, if need be, persons more legally trained, referred to as legally authorized representatives (LAR), may also be required to participate in the informed consent process.

This proposal was further complicated by the distinction between research projects with only minimal risk and those with more significant risk for the patient. The requirements in each case are sufficiently different that they add to the difficulties imposed on the smooth functioning of important research projects. For example, if the research involves no greater than minimal risks, the following actions must be taken: First, if the subject is able to consent to participate in the project, the giving of consent would be monitored by a consent advocate, and any patient objection to entering into the study would have to be honored by the researchers. Second, if the patient cannot consent, then the IRB must be shown how the research project relates to the patient's condition. The patient must also be able to "assent" (i.e., know the difference between "yes" and "no") and not object to the experimental treatment. The IRB would appoint a consent advocate who, along with a LAR, must consent to allow participation of the patient. The requirements are different if the patient is unable to consent or object, or if the risk is greater than minimal. In this case, other considerations apply, such as the extent of direct benefit to the patient and the importance of the research for societal betterment.

These proposed 1978 regulations indicate that obtaining informed consent may require considerable administrative activity. Even though these regulations have not been approved in their proposed form, they remain important. They will continue to affect policy regarding the mentally disabled as they address some of the concerns society has about the "competency" of patients to give informed consent and, therefore, to control what happens to them in research projects or therapy.

Final regulations amending the basic policy of the then Department of Health and Human Services (HHS) were published in January 1981 (Final Regulations, 1981). Specific regulations protecting the institutionalized mentally disabled have not yet been developed. With regard to general research concerns, these regulations incorporate some of the provisions proposed by the National Commission but essentially disregard the various levels of patient competence and exempt from IRB review research that presents little or no risk of harm to the subject. Furthermore, certain categories of research that involve no more than "minimal risk" may proceed after expedited review by the appropriate IRB. (See Final Regulations, 1981; Tancredi & Maxfield, 1983.)

Informed Consent in the Treatment Setting

Several landmark cases relate to the issue of informed consent in the context of therapy, particularly *Cobbs v. Grant* (1972) and *Canterbury v. Spense* (1972). The jury decisions in these cases enhanced the patient's power by considering whether treatment information not provided by the physician might have been of such import as to materially influence the patient's decision. The juries took the position that, had the risks been fully disclosed, a prudent and reasonable person might not have consented to the recommended therapy. This is an "objective" test, which approaches materiality of risk from the "reasonable man" standpoint as opposed to the "subjective" test specific to a particular patient, applied in the case of *McPherson v. Ellis* (1982). In general, then, the test for determining what information should be disclosed was based on the extent to which the information would have materially affected a patient's consent. Though the cited cases do not specify how much information should be disclosed or provide precise guidelines for patients, they nonetheless have had a widespread effect in various jurisdictions.

Other cases, however, have maintained the philosophy that the physician should have some privilege over the information to be disclosed where full disclosure may be detrimental to the patient's welfare and preclude a reasoned decision (*Karp v. Cooley*, 1972). Also, there are obvious exemptions to informed consent, for example, in case of emergency or when a patient voluntarily waives the right to participate in informed consent decisions. And, if a patient is judged incompetent, the decision may be left to a next of kin or judicial determination.

Though the objectives of informed consent seem reasonable, that is, to diminish the arbitrary paternalism and the force of the authority model, both so pervasive in the health care system, and, as much as possible, to shift decision making onto the patient, considerable debate has challenged whether informed consent is only a theoretically rather than practically sound concept. It seems to many to give verbal attention to patient values but insufficient protection on a pragmatic level. This point rests on two factors: First, even with all essential information, the patient will have limited understanding and ultimately rely on the physician's judgment; second, the physician's predisposition will influence the way the information is presented and bias the patient toward (or away from) particular treatment options.

In addition to the requirements described in the HHS guidelines for informed consent, such as the kind of information that should be presented on benefits, risks, and alternatives, other considerations enter into determining whether informed consent is valid. These considerations were first articulated in a case involving the use of psychosurgery for controlling violent behavior (*Kaimowitz v. Michigan Department of Mental Hygiene*, 1973). Three elements were defined as important in a meaningful informed consent: "voluntariness" of the consent, competence of the consenter, and materiality of the information provided by the physician. These elements are important ultimately, because they address the fairness of informed consent. Voluntariness refers to the extent to which the individual is free to make a decision. Institutionalized persons such as mental patients, the retarded, and prisoners may not be in the best position to provide voluntary consent. For example, the use of prisoners with mental disability would raise questions about motivation. The argument might be made that the prisoners saw an opportunity for possible early release or minimizing the onerousness of their stay in the institution, so that their participation was not quite "voluntary." Similarly, mentally disturbed or disabled individuals are under the influence of the value system of mental health institutions and may also enter into a research project to gain certain advantages in that system.

Competence to consent is a particularly difficult issue to deal with in research and therapy involving the mentally ill and retarded. It implies a capacity to understand the nature and consequences of their decision, including an awareness of the risks, benefits, and available alternatives. As already discussed with respect to proposed guidelines on research involving the mentally ill (Protection of Human Subjects, 1978), two levels of "competency" have been described: "assent" and "consent." The issue of competence is highly pertinent also to research on children and the elderly.

The materiality of the information to be made available to the patient is perhaps one of the most problematic concerns in informed consent. One may argue that research into a certain treatment is at such an early stage that data are inadequate to help form any reasonable estimate of benefits, risks, and alternatives. When this is the case, even though the patient is given all available information and voluntarily and competently agrees to enter into the research project, the materiality of the information can be judged so insufficient that it precludes truly informed consent. Unfortunately, the Kaimowitz case does not provide useful guidelines for recognizing when information exceeds a threshold level of materiality so that informed consent is possible. On the other hand, the idea of materiality of information does introduce a very important consideration in that it emphasizes the merits of well-designed clinical trials for assessing the effectiveness of diagnostic and treatment modalities. A concern with materiality of information is a concern with the uncertainty of results in an area where consequences can be debilitating if not life-threatening. It promotes an appreciation that well-designed studies are essential for creating the data base that raises information above the desired threshold of materiality.

An important question that often comes up is whether or not the risks of new and experimental technology are generally greater than those of traditional therapies for particular diseases. The answer has bearing on the extent to which society should be tolerant of human experimentation. The main study on experimental risks was conducted by Gilbert et al. (1977), who examined 46 journal papers that dealt with randomized clinical trials in anesthesiology and surgery and involved at least 10 patients per trial. In their investigations the researchers demonstrated that it is a fallacious belief that new therapies necessarily create higher risks. They showed that approximately half the therapeutic innovations tested by randomized clinical trials resulted in some improvements for the patient, and approximately 24 percent reduced complications. Their conclusion was that persons in the experimental groups were not much better or worse off than those in the control, or traditional therapy, groups. An inference from their conclusion is that when physicians have felt intuitively before conducting trials, that an experimental treatment may be better than the traditional treatment, then these advance expectations have not tended to cause patient injuries in either the experimental or control group. This study is important because it dealt directly with the ethical propriety of dividing patients into experimental and control groups in randomized clinical trials, particularly when the research physicians have a medical preference for one type of treatment over another. Certainly in the analysis of investigations in anesthesiology and surgery, it appears that on balance the net gain or loss from innovative treatments over traditional therapies is near zero.

The discussion thus far has dealt with difficulties in using the concept of informed consent to provide protection for patients in the medical care system. Now consider three categories of concerns basic to the problems of applying the concept of informed consent to research with medical and psychiatric patients.

Patient Competence

The question of competence refers to the patient's ability to comprehend information provided by physicians or other experimenters. One can readily understand that patients overwhelmed by emergency conditions, such as acute suffering, are less likely to fully comprehend information they are given about proposed treatment. However, even less stressful, nonemergency situations can adversely affect comprehension. Only a few studies have really attempted to grapple with the problem of the competence of patients, even of average intelligence and emotional stability, to comprehend medical information. One such study (Cassileth et al., 1980) involved an evaluation of the ability of cancer patients to recall information given them on consent forms with regard to the use of chemotherapy, radiation therapy, or surgery. The day after they signed the forms consenting to treatment, 200 patients filled out questionnaires designed to determine their levels of understanding and their opinions about the purpose of the documents they had signed. Of this group, 60 percent demonstrated that they understood the nature and purpose of the treatments; 35 percent were able to identify at least one possible major complication of treatment; and only 40 percent showed they had actually read the forms carefully. Most of the patients seemed to scan the forms quickly and to rely mostly on what their physicians told them.

The authors of the study suggested three factors that may be responsible for the patients' difficulties. First, ability to recall seemed somewhat associated with the patients' medical conditions. Ambulatory patients seemed to do significantly better than those who were bedridden. Second, and not too surprising, was an apparent direct relationship between educational background and the capacity to read and comprehend the medical information. Third, the patients' perceptions of the forms correlated with the care with which they read the material and their level of recall.

Another study (Grundner, 1980), of the readability of forms for consent for surgery, suggested that other factors, specifically the language used in the forms, may help to explain patients' problems in understanding medical information. This study showed that the forms were difficult to comprehend, even after careful reading, by those with adequate education. The obvious conclusion is that the profession has a major responsibility not only to provide information but to do so in a form that at least the average, educated, concerned patient can comprehend.

The study on the comprehension by cancer patients of the side effects and benefits of the three major cancer therapies dealt with problems of the competence to make decisions of normal patients not suffering from mental or emotional disabilities. Only a few studies have dealt with mental patients who voluntarily agreed to enter a treatment program. The two such studies briefly described below involved patients who were in a position to volunteer, which suggests that, for the most part, their psychiatric conditions were not serious enough to require involuntary hospitalization. In one of the studies (Palmer & Wohl, 1972), only 8 were rated as fully informed of the terms of their voluntary admission.

The second study (Olin & Olin, 1975) involved interviewing 40 patients regarding their understanding of three forms typically filled out when a patient volunteers to enter a hospital: the information release form, the legal rights form, and the voluntary admissions form. Twenty were interviewed between one and three days after admission, and 20 were interviewed seven to ten days after admission. Twenty-eight demonstrated the ability to fully comprehend all three forms. Twelve were unable to read at least one of the forms—especially the permission for information release—but understood the other two. Two patients could not understand the voluntary admission form but could read the other two forms. There seemed to be some relation between the length of hospital stay and the patients ability to comprehend the three forms, probably reflecting the fact that the longer the patients were in the hospital, the more likely they were to learn the information from other patients and staff.

Though these studies involved a relatively small group of patients, they point to the formidable difficulties of obtaining informed consent from patients suffering from diseased conditions that directly affect their capacity to understand information and arrive at a rational decision. Grossman & Summers (1980) suggested that very few schizophrenics may be able to give the fully informed consent required by law. But, as already mentioned, not only the mentally ill present problems of consent. Others include the mentally retarded, children, and the elderly suffering from organic brain dysfunction. The importance of the two studies of mental patients and the one of cancer patients is that they demonstrate, in many respects, that informed consent may be more fiction than fact as a protective device for patients, even patients who are intellectually and emotionally sound enough to comprehend the medical information presented to them. This dissonance between the information presented and a patient's comprehension of it is augmented by the fact that the information may be presented in a way that causes the physician's personal preferences to dominate and affect the patient's decisions.

Judgment under Uncertainty

The second main issue that affects the meaningfulness of informed consent concerns the making of judgments under conditions of uncertainty. Even if the physician provides all necessary information, and the patient is able to understand and assimilate it, danger is still inherent in making choices under conditions of uncertainty. In their classic article on this topic, Tversky & Kahneman (1974) claimed that people faced with choices that are not obvious fall back into a circumscribed number of heuristic principles that operate relatively automatically, thus avoiding the complicated task of deciphering the probabilities of benefits and risks in a specific decision. These heuristic principles, which underlie many of our decisions, can often be useful but may also sometimes result in serious errors of judgment. The tendency to rely on heuristic principles is by no means limited to laymen, or to those who are mentally dysfunctional, but can be experienced by experts in their fields.

Tversky & Kahneman referred to three general heuristic principles used by decision-makers to predict the outcome of particular choices. All three work against the paying of sufficient attention to realistic probabilities in decision-making and expose many of the fallacies that can occur in reliance on intuitive judgment alone. The first principle is called *representativeness*. Representativeness means that there is insensitivity to the probability of outcomes, including prior probabilities. This is created by the fact that one event, A, may be linked to another, B, simply because they resemble each other or may appear similar to the decision maker. For example, if a patient is confronted with the proposed use of a new psychoactive drug, and the physician describes it in such a way that the patient feels it resembles an already familiar drug, say Thorazine, then the patient may expect the new drug to have benefits and side effects similar to those of Thorazine. Objectively, the data on the new drug may indicate a significantly greater probability of side effects. Nevertheless, the influence of the action of representativeness may distort the results, rendering them insensitive to sample size and creating misconceptions as to the effects of chance, regression, and unpredictability. By ignoring factual information about probability and unpredictability, the patient may overestimate or underestimate the effects of the new drug due to association with the drug it ostensibly "resembles." The second heuristic principle, called *adjustment* and *anchoring*, refers to the use of an initial value as an anchor or basis for estimates that are adjusted in order to arrive at a final conclusion. The anchor point is essentially intuitive, and the subsequent adjustments inevitably bias the evaluation of events. The third principle is *availability*, which refers to the estimate of probabilities on the basis of the ease with which similar occurrences can be brought to the mind of the decision maker. The ability to recall and imagine similar incidents will bias expectations of the effects of the new decision.

Though these heuristic principles are economic and effective in a variety of circumstances because they allow quick response without complete analysis, they also serve the important psychodynamic function of allowing some denial of anxiety-provoking uncertainty. In the case of new technologies or drug developments, these heuristic principles can distort perceptions of how these innovations may function in a total system of health care, preclude proper assessment of the influence of human error, and create overconfidence in available scientific and medical knowledge of the developments (Slovic et al., 1979; Star 1980).

The fact that one has expert knowledge of science and medicine does not mean that heuristic principles will not be employed in the face of uncertainty. For example, a study (Bunker & Brown, 1974) was done to determine whether surgical services are overused because uninformed consumers overestimate their benefits. The investigators compared the use of surgical and anesthesiological services by physicians and their families with the use by other professionals such as lawyers. The rates for physicians and their spouses was found in some cases to be as much as 25 to 30 percent higher than for the general population of professionals. This suggests that knowledgeable consumers, such as physicians, place a high value on the benefits to be achieved through surgical services. However, two operations, hysterectomies and appendectomies, which have come under considerable criticism in recent years, were particularly prevalent. It was estimated from the observed rate that more than half of the wives of physicians were likely to have a hysterectomy by the time they reached 65 years of age.

The fact that these operations are of questionable merit in a large majority of cases seems to support the Tversky & Kahneman contention that reliance on heuristic principles may result in considerable errors of judgment. To a large extent it is understandable that physicians tend to seek medical intervention, even when the recommended surgery may not be effective, because of the long conditioning they receive in medical school, internship, and residency. It may also be true that, even though operations such as hysterectomies, appendectomies, and colectomies may be minimally effective in the vast majority of cases, when they are recommended to a physician they have a special appeal because heuristic principles find a fertile ground in someone professionally active in the treatment of disease. An example in the field of psychiatry would be the tendency of residents who work with patients requiring lithium carbonate and who are doing research on manic depression, to fit every new patient into one of the already familiar categories. Thus, a judgment distorted by the heuristic principles may lead to a misdiagnosis of a seriously paranoid schizophrenic or a patient suffering from some organic mental syndrome.

Impact of Placebo Effect

The last and perhaps most difficult problem with informed consent involves the placebo effect (Levine et al., 1978), the enhancement of therapeutic results by the patient's favorable belief and expectations, even in the absence of any known, objective relationship between the therapy and the condition being treated. The classical placebo effect is a benefit a patient received from a nonactive agent.

An interesting illustration of how the placebo effect can distort the results of even active treatments is provided by a study (Benson & McCallie, 1979; Kolata, 1980) evaluating five abandoned treatments for angina pectoris: Zanthines, Khellen, vitamin E, ligation of the internal mammary artery, and implantation of that artery. Each was at one time or other considered the most effective treatment for angina pectoris. Although much of the work that later refuted the value of these treatments was not conducted through double-blind randomized clinical trials, a characteristic pattern was revealed. In each case, when the treatments were introduced, initial studies showed an effectiveness of 70 to 90 percent. Benson & McCallie had labeled the earlier investigators "enthusiasts" because they firmly believed in the effectiveness of the treatments they were testing. A few years after each treatment was acclaimed, it was either displaced by one of the other four or retested by more skeptical researchers who found its effectiveness to be only 30 to 40 percent, no greater than the baseline level expected from a placebo. In the conclusion drawn from these contradictions, it was suggested that the beliefs and expectations of the physician in the early stages of therapy spill over to the patients and create the placebo effect. As newer treatments were introduced, and more skeptical physicians became involved in the studies, the placebo effect, and the observed benefits of the treatment, diminished.

The placebo effect, the influence of heuristic principles, and the issue of patient competence must all be considered because they can affect validity and meaningfulness of informed consent as a protective device for the patient. Even if all material information about a treatment is made available, and the patient is capable (i.e., competent) of comprehending the medical facts and arriving at an unfettered consent, a true assessment of treatment benefits, risks, and alternatives may be precluded by the placebo effect and the action of heuristic principles. Hence, for a study to be accurate, it may have to include a means of factoring out the placebo effect. Ethical considerations may also have to be taken into account in the use of the placebo in experimentation. Many scholars argue strongly that placebo controls in randomized clinical trials constitute deception in medical practice (Simmons, 1978). Sissela Bok (Bok, 1974) recommended that certain principles be adopted for use of the placebo, including obligating the experimenter to respond honestly to patients who ask if a placebo is to be used in their care, and an absolute prohibition against giving placebos if patients explicitly object to them or if other treatments for the patient's condition are clearly indicated.

Nonmedical Information

Another question affecting informed consent is the nature and extent of what might be called "nonmedical" information that should be provided patients exposed to clinical experimentation or treatment. Such information goes beyond expected benefits and risks and concerns matters like the variation of treatment effectiveness with the particular health care setting. With regard to surgery, for example, a study by Luft et al. (1979) showed that a hospital's success rate for a given procedure varied significantly with the number of such procedures performed per year. Specifically, the mortality rates for open heart surgery, vascular surgery, transurethral resection of the prostate, and coronary bypass surgery in hospitals that performed 200 or more of each of these procedure were 25 to 41 percent lower than in hospitals that performed substantially fewer such procedures. Of course, for some less complicated surgical procedures, such as total hip replacement and total cholecystectomy, the study showed little difference between hospitals of high and low volume. Nonetheless, the study demonstrated the important fact that success rates can depend on hospital experience. This reflects not only the hospitals' different abilities to deal adequately with the surgical procedure itself but different levels of crucial pre- and postoperative supportive patient care.

Thus, in psychiatry it is quite conceivable that clinics or hospitals that treat large numbers of manic-depressive patients with lithium carbonate, or severely depressed patients with electroshock treatments, are likely to achieve better results and incur less morbidity than those with less experience. Such comparative studies, between major academic centers and smaller community facilities, for example, have not been done routinely for new technological developments in psychiatric practice but seem ethically necessary to provide health care consumers with information they should have. The Luft, Bunker, & Enthoven study confirmed what many have felt for some time, that success rate, morbidity, and mortality differ in different settings. This obligates health care providers to conduct similar studies for the full range of medical and psychiatric services offered by their institutions. For those engaged in a research study, it is also ethically appropriate that information about the success rates of those conducting the study, even for the administration of traditional therapies, be made available to patients before they participate in the study.

Another area not yet important in the field of psychiatry but with tremendous potential in the future, is the use of algorithms for so-called routine care. In medical and surgical services, techniques such as criteria mapping are being increasingly used to deal with the signs and symptoms of a wide variety of conditions (Greenfield et al., 1977; Greenfield & Jordan, 1978). Various studies have shown that protocols for evaluating the significance of symptoms such as chest pain and signs of lymphadenopathy are very effective. These protocols work by involving a group of nonphysicians or, in the case of psychiatry, psychiatric mental health professionals, who manage the patient through a pre-established decision-making logic, which may include a series of evaluative tests and procedures. In psychiatry, when patients enter a hospital complaining of hallucinations or forgetfulness, it should be relatively easy to place them in a protocol of interviews and tests handled by mental health professionals, after the steps have been previously delineated by psychiatrists, who have the expertise in the differential diagnosis of mental diseases. This does raise the ethical concern that patients who enter a system of criteria mapping may be put through all the tests even though in any one case it might be argued that not all the tests are necessary. The mere application of an algorithm may channel patients through the entire protocol. These diagnostic procedures may sometimes entail risks, not to mention increased costs for the patient. Furthermore, as the use of algorithms or criteria mapping becomes more prevalent in the health care system, in psychiatry in particular, it is possible that they will be used for more complex signs and symptoms. Although this innovation is not yet a major component of psychiatric practice it may become so because it could more efficiently use paraprofessionals—nurses, clinicians, phy-

sicians' assistants, and clinical social workers—in the mental
health field.

In addition to the problems of technology assessment and
information disclosure in the design of epidemiological studies,
particularly with regard to protecting the patient or subject in research, two other areas of ethical concern in psychiatric epidemiology must be considered—confidentiality of information
and the right to refuse treatment—which affect, directly or indirectly, the appropriateness of various research studies. Since
each of these topics could require an extensive analysis in its
own right, this discussion will briefly focus on those issues most
relevant to psychiatric epidemiology.

Patient Confidentiality

There has been growing concern about the confidentiality of
information, particularly in regard to access to patient records.
In 1974, the Privacy Act imposed major impediments on access
to records without explicit patient permission. Unfortunately,
this and similar laws that created difficulties in obtaining records
had a major obstructive impact on research, particularly longitudinal studies requiring more detailed information about patients
to assess a range of personal characteristics, such as those that
might relate to the development of mental and emotional disabilities (Robins, 1978). Of course there was also a major need to
increase the protection of personal information due to incursions by third party payers and agencies for psychiatric information to judge the necessity of treatment and the quality of care.

In recognition of the competing societal needs of privacy of
personal information and the benefits of well-devised longitudinal and other epidemiological studies, the Privacy Protection
Study Commission was established in 1975 by Congress to review the appropriate role of federal regulation with respect to
privacy. In 1977 the Commission produced its report which examined the confidentiality of medical care records with particular regard to the use of these records for biomedical and epidemiological research (U.S. Privacy Protection Commission,
1977). The Commission concluded that individual subjects need
more protection from inadvertent disclosure of information by
administrative actions, but also recognized that statistical and

epidemiological research into various diagnostic and treatment methods is vital to public welfare.

The Commission was particularly concerned about identifiers that could provide easy access to personal information. It agreed that records should be made available for research purposes but took a strong position that subjects of research must be notified if the information obtained may possibly be used for additional research or other statistical purposes, and that it not be in a form that is individually identifiable. The Commission also took the position that a patient must be informed if the information in an identifiable form is to be disclosed for purposes other than research. It further asserted that any agency may disclose identifiable information without obtaining patient consent if the agency determines that the information is necessary to accomplish the research purpose. However, the agency must first determine that the importance of the statistical research is significant enough to warrant the risk of subjecting the individual to additional exposure. Hence, the agency disclosing the information must devise a balancing test to establish that the social benefit to be achieved warrants incursions on individual privacy. Even so, adequate safeguards are required to protect records from unnecessary disclosure, for example, means for removing or destroying identifiers.

Epidemiological studies, particularly longitudinal studies that follow patients over a long period of time, require closer vigilance and more patient information than a simple survey. To check all possible factors in morbidity and mortality risks may even require examination of employment and other personal records of patients for clues to the origins of stress or other contributions to a disease condition. For example, Occupational Safety and Health Administration regulations (OSHA, 1980) give OSHA access to personally identifiable employee exposure and medical records. Since research is usually interested in large groups exposed to similar conditions, rather than in individuals, the revealing of more personal data should not result in infractions of confidentiality. However researchers should certainly be held to the highest level of responsibility and obligation for maintaining the personal privacy of records and for destroying identifiers and other revealing notations as soon as they are no longer necessary for research. The problems of confidentiality in longitudinal studies and other epidemiological research have not been totally resolved, but the Commission recommendations, by promoting a balance between the benefits to society and the risks of individual patient disclosures, take a big step toward recognizing that it is possible to achieve both ends in broad-scale research whose objectives in obtaining personal information are statistical assessment rather than acquiring possibly detrimental information about individuals (U.S. Privacy Protection Commission, 1977).

Somewhat related to the issue of confidentiality is the problem posed by the landmark case of *Tarasoff v. The Regents of the University of California* (1976). The court's decision, which held that a psychotherapist has an affirmative obligation to protect (warn) potential victims against possible injury by a dangerous patient, may create conflicts and obligations for the epidemiological researcher. For example, it is conceivable that a project may involve subjects who are violence-prone. If the *Tarasoff* decision applies (although the original jurisdiction was California, other states such as New Jersey, have had similar cases—see *McIntosh v. Milano*, 1979), the researcher would be obligated to warn where appropriate. This would require a more intimate relationship between a researcher and individuals who display a high tendency toward violence, as well as a determination of possible victims. Beyond the legal obligation is the ethical question that arises when a researcher is aware of a potentially dangerous individual and a likely victim. Even though confidentiality may possibly be compromised, the philosophical basis underlying *Tarasoff* is rather compelling, that is, we do live in a risk-taking society and, to whatever extent possible, have some obligation to minimize that risk. (Some more recent cases seem to be addressing more explicitly and extending the concept of "protect" in *Tarasoff*—see *Jablonski v. U.S.*, 1983, and *Lipari v. Sears Roebuck and Company*, 1980).

There has been considerable debate on the impact of *Tarasoff* on psychotherapy, some arguing that a duty to warn has had a chilling effect. Although there have been no really good studies on this issue, the *Stanford Law Review* (California Survey: *Tarasoff*, 1978) suggested that some of the detrimental effects of *Tarasoff* manifest themselves as increased time devoted during psychotherapy to ferreting out patients' propensities for violence, uneasiness on the part of the therapist (e.g., anxiety over legal obligations), playing it safe by mislabeling increasing numbers of patients as potentially dangerous, and an incentive to turn away patients with homicidal tendencies. Psychiatric epidemiological research may be similarly affected in jurisdictions where *Tarasoff* applies, particularly in the avoidance of gathering information on violence-potential that would obligate the researchers to warn possible victims.

Right to Refuse Treatment

HHS guidelines explicitly uphold the right of patients participating in clinical experimentation to request termination of involvement with no prejudice to appropriate therapy. Hence, for example, patients receiving experimental drugs for endogenous depression would have the prerogative, as part of the research requirements, to leave the study without prejudicing other proper treatment by the health care institution (Protection of Human Research Subjects, 1979, 1981; Protection of Human Subjects, 1978). Cases on the right to refuse treatment, like *Rogers v. Okin* (1979), *Rogers v. Commissioner of the Department of Mental Health* (1983), and *Rennie v. Klein* (1979, 1983), focus particularly on the involuntarily committed psychiatric patient who is *not deemed incompetent* by the courts to refuse psychotropic medication. In *Rogers v. Okin* this right applied absolutely to involuntarily committed mental patients who have not been adjudicated incompetent except for periods of an emergency, i.e., an imminent threat of harm to self or others, or to prevent irreversible and substantial deterioration. (In the case of incompetent patients this right must be exercised through "substituted" judgment.) During these times, the staff may medicate these patients against their will. In *Rennie v. Klein* the final decision maker on the right of an involuntarily committed, dangerous, mentally ill patient to refuse psychotropic medication is the medical director or the director's designee. Such action is judged necessary to prevent the patient from doing harm to self or others.

It is important to consider the impact of these decisions on research that deals with a large number of involuntarily committed patients in an acute psychotic state. According to decisions like *Rogers v. Okin*, such patients may, upon recuperating from an acute disturbance, refuse psychotropic medications. For example, a study examining the long-term therapeutic effects of a neuroleptic on schizophrenia must take into account that these patients, once recuperated from the acute stage, may refuse the medication. Such interruption may distort the outcome of the research.

The obverse of the right of psychiatric patients to refuse psychotropic medication is the obligation of the researcher to adequately diagnose and treat those discovered during the study to have serious disease. For illustration, a study assessing the diagnostic validity of parameters for evaluating schizo-affective schizophrenia may turn up a small percentage of cases of the control population who suffer from this condition. The researchers then have an obligation to provide adequate follow-up and, if need be, channel these individuals into an appropriate therapeutic program. Patients entering into research projects, therefore, not only have a right to refuse treatment at any point during the course of the study but also, by participating, obligate the researchers to provide access to care for those discovered to have serious diseases.

Conclusion

This discussion of technology assessment and ethical considerations in psychiatric epidemiology has concentrated on three major areas. First, the design and scientific validity of the studies must be suitably evaluated in advance, with emphasis on the importance of randomized clinical trials, statistically adequate numbers of patients and appropriate counting procedures, and awareness of the frailties of nonrandomized studies as they affect the scientific accuracy of results. The discussion also dealt with the ethical obligations of the profession to conduct appropriate effectiveness studies of primary modalities of treatment and to adhere to well-defined guidelines for accurate studies. The Fletcher analysis of studies published in the major medical journals, *JAMA*, *Lancet*, and the *New England Journal of Medicine*, examined the strengths and weaknesses of research design and showed that research designs tended to become weaker during the 1970s. This places a burden on the profession to carefully examine in its scientific journals the statistical and epidemiological accuracy of the research studies being reported.

Second, attention was given to the power prerogatives of patients and physicians, with particular emphasis on information disclosure requirements, competence, the influences of heuristic judgments and the conceptual difficulties posed by the ill-defined placebo effect.

Last, in keeping with an examination of the power prerogatives in the therapeutic relationship, two important issues—confidentiality and the right to refuse treatment—were briefly discussed. Increasing sensitivity to the egregious disclosure of private patient information has begun to stimulate legislative proposals for further protecting this important property right of consumers. Studies relying on demographic and medical parameters must take into account the requirements of confidentiality of information. The right to refuse treatment and the obligation of researchers to channel into proper treatment those discovered to have serious illnesses again emphasize the increasing rights of patients used for experimental purposes (Title VIII, California Administrative Code, 1980). It is important also to cite the increasing concern about informing patients before they enter studies what obligations the institutions or researchers will assume in medical care and consequent losses should injury occur. For some time, many have been proposing a no-fault system of compensation for those injured in the course of human experimentation, but it has not yet become a reality in the requirements of the Department of Health and Human Services (formerly the Department of Health, Education and Welfare) and its guidelines.

The ethics of psychiatric epidemiology is also concerned with assuring that adequate medical care information is made available to consumers and patients. Underlying this discussion is the presupposition articulated in A. L. Cochran's classic work, (Cochran, 1972) that an absolute obligation exists for the profession to subject its diagnostic and therapeutic methods to efficacy and efficiency studies. As was pointed out earlier by Luft, Bunker, & Enthoven (1979), significant differences exist in morbidity and mortality rates for various procedures not only among practitioners but among different care settings. It is, therefore, mandatory that comparative studies of diagnostic and therapeutic results be conducted to provide consumers with the best available information upon which to make a decision, not only about accepting therapeutic options offered by physicians but about agreeing to procedures in specific care settings. As indicated by the review of studies on randomized clinical trials and technology assessment, much can be learned from those areas of medical care that have long been sensitive to the importance of clinical trials and statistical techniques. Clearly, the psychiatric care of patients has to be rendered with the same degree of scientific rigor and accuracy applied to studies and research on serious mental illness.

References

Benson, H. & McCallie, D. P., Jr. (1979), Angina pectoris and the placebo effect. *N. Engl. J. Med.* 300:1424–1429.

Bok, S. (1974), The ethics of giving placebos. *Scientific American* 231: 17–23.

Boncheck, L. I. (1979), Are randomized trials appropriate for evaluating new operations? *N. Engl. J. Med.* 301:44–45.

Bunker, J. P., Barnes, B. A., & Mosteller, F. (1977), *Cost, Risks and Benefits of Surgery*, p. 308. New York: Oxford University Press.

Bunker, J. P. & Brown, B. W. (1974), The physician-patient as an informed consumer of surgical services. *N. Engl. J. Med.* 290:1051–1055.

Byar, D. P. et al. (1976), Randomized clinical trials. *N. Engl. J. Med.* 295:74–79.

California Survey (1978), *Tarasoff. Stanford Law Review* 31:165.

Canterbury v. Spence (1972), 464 F. 2d 772 (D.C.).

Cassileth, B. R., Zupkis, R. V., & Sutton-Smith, K. (1980), Informed consent—Why are its goals imperfectly realized? *N. Engl. J. Med.* 302:896–899.

Cobbs v. Grant (1972), 8 Cal. 3d 229, 104 Cal. RPTR 505, 502 P. 2d 1.

Cochran, A. L. (1972), *Effectiveness and Efficiency: Random Reflections on Health Services.* London: Burgess and Sons.

Fletcher, R. H. & Fletcher, S. W. (1979), Clinical research in general medical journals—A thirty year perspective. *N. Engl. J. Med.* 301: 180–183.

Frazer, H. S. & Hiatt, H. H. (1978), Evaluation of medical practices. *Science* 200:875–878.

Freiman, J. A., Chalmers, T. C., Smith, H., Jr., et al. (1978), The importance of beta, the type two error and sample size in the design and interpretation of the randomized clinical trial. *N. Engl. J. Med.* 299: 690–694.

Gahen, E. A. & Freireich, E. J. (1974), Non-randomized controls in cancer clinical trials. *N. Engl. J. Med.* 290:198–203.

Gilbert, J. P., McPeek, B., & Mostellar, F. (1977), Statistics and ethics in surgery and anesthesia. *Science* 198:684–689.

Goldzieher, A. et al. (1971), A placebo controlled double-blind, cross-over investigation of side effects attributed to all contraceptives. *J. Fertil. Steril.* 22:609–623.

Greenfield, S. et al. (1977), The clinical investigation and measurement of chest pain in an emergency department. *Medical Care* 15:898–905.

Greenfield, S. & Jordan, C. (1978), The clinical investigation of lymphadenopathy in primary care practice. *J. Am. Med. Assoc.* 240:1388–1393.

Grossman, L. & Summers, F. (1980), A study of the capacity of schizophrenic patients to give informed consent. *Hosp. Community Psychiatry* 31:205.

Grundner, T. M. (1980), On the readability of surgical consent forms. *N. Engl. J. Med.* 302:900–902.

Jablonski v. U.S. (1983), 712 F. 2d 391.

Kaimowitz v. Michigan Department of Mental Hygiene (1973), Cir. Ct. Wayne County, Michigan, unreported.

Karp v. Cooley (1972), 349 F. Supp. 827.

Kolata, G. B. (1980), Dilemma in cancer treatment. *Science* 209:792–794. "Desire to believe in cancer therapy is so profound that people don't want to hear the disbelievers."

Levine, J. B., Gordon, N. C., & Fields, H. L. (1978), The mechanism of placebo analgesia. *Lancet,* September 23:654–657.

Lipari v. Sears Roebuck and Company (1980), 497 F. Supp. 185 (DC Neb.).

Luft, H. S., Bunker, J. P., & Enthoven, A. C. (1979), Should operations be regionalized? *N. Engl. J. Med.* 301:1364–1369.

McIntosh v. Milano (1979), 403 A. 2d 500.

McPherson v. Ellis (1982), 287 S.E. 2d 896 (N.C.).

Mather, H. G., Morgan, D. C., Pearson, N. G., et al. (1976), Myocardial infarction: A comparison between home and hospital care for patients. *Br. Med. J.* 8:925–929.

Mather, H. G., Pearson, N. G., Read, K. L., et al. (1971), Acute myocardial infarction: Home and hospital treatment. *Br. Med. J.* 3:334–338.

Meisel, A. (1979), The "exceptions" to the informed consent doctrine: Striking a balance between competing values in medical decision making. *Wisconsin Law Review* 1979:413–488.

Murphy, M. L., Holtgren, H. N., Detre, K., et al. (1977), Treatment of chronic stable angina: A preliminary report of survival data of the randomized Veterans Administration comparative study. *N. Engl. J. Med.* 297(12):621–627.

Occupational Safety and Health Administration (OSHA) Regulations (1980), *Federal Register* 45:35277.

Olin, G. B. & Olin, H. S. (1975), Informed consent in voluntary mental hospital admissions. *Am. J. Psychiatry* 132:938–941.

Palmer, A. B. & Wohl, J. (1972), Voluntary admission forms: Does the patient know what he is signing? *Hosp. Community Psychiatry* 23: 250–252.

Park, L. C. et al. (1967), Effects of informed consent on research patients study results. J. *Nerv. Ment. Dis.* 145:349–357.

Protection of Human Research Subjects, DHEW (FDA) (1979), *Federal Register* 44:47696–47697.

————, Final regulations amending basic HHS policy for the protection of human research subjects (1981), *Federal Register* 46:8366–8391.

Protection of Human Subjects (1978), Proposed regulations on research involving those institutionalized as mentally disabled. *Federal Register* 43:53950–53956.

Rennie v. Klein (1979), 476 F. Supp. 1294 (D. N.J.).

———— (1983), 720 F. 2d 266 (3d Cir.) (en banc).

Report and Recommendations of the National Commission for the Protection of Human Subjects of Biomedical and Behavioral Research: Institutional Review Boards (1978), *Federal Register* 43:56175.

Robins, L. N. (1978), The consequences of the recommendations of the Privacy Protection Study Commission for Longitudinal Studies. Address presented at the Life History Research and Psychopathology meeting, Cincinnati.

Rogers v. Commissioner of the Department of Mental Health (1983), 390 Mass. 489 (Mass. Sup. Jud. Ct.).

Rogers v. Okin (1979), 478 F. Supp. 1342.

———— (1984), 738F. 2d 1.

Sackett, D. L. & Gent, N. (1979), Controversy in counting and attributing events in clinical trials. *N. Engl. J. Med.* 301:1410–1413.

Salgo v. Leland Stanford, Jr., University Board of Trustees (1957), 154 Cal. App. 2d 560, 317 P. 2d 170.

Simmons, B. (1978), Problems in deceptive medical procedures: An ethical and legal analysis of the administration of placebo. *J. Med. Ethics* 4:172–181.

Slovic, P., Fischoff, G., Lichtenstein, S. (1979), Rating and risks. *Environment* 21:14–39.

Star, C. (1980), Risks and risk decisions. *Science* 108:1114–1119.

Tancredi, L. R. & Maxfield, C. T. (1983), Regulation of psychiatric research: A socioethical analysis. *Int. J. Law Psychiatry*, 6:17–38.

Tancredi, L. R. & Slaby, A. E. (1977), *Ethical Policy in Mental Health Care: The Goals of Psychiatric Intervention.* New York: Neale Watson.

Tarasoff v. The Regents of the University of California (1976), 551 P. 2d 334.

Title VIII California Administrative Code, §859 X.C. (1980), California's adoption of new administrative regulations relating to the right of voluntary patients to refuse anti-psychotic medications. *Mental Disability Law Reporter*, May 4. (This is one example of state legislative changes on the right to refuse psychotropic medication.)

Tukey, J. W. (1977), Some thoughts on clinical trials, especially problems of multiplicity. *Science* 198:679–683.

Tversky, H. & Kahneman, D. (1974), Judgment under uncertainty: Heuristic and biases. *Science* 185:1124–1136.

U.S. Privacy Protection Commission (1977), *The Report of the Privacy Protection Study Commission.* Washington, D.C.: U.S. Government Printing Office.

Zelen, M. (1979), A new design for randomized clinical trials. *N. Engl. J. Med.* 300:1242–1245.

Chapter 2

Diagnostic Ethics:
The Uses and Limits of
Psychiatric Explanation*

WALTER REICH

Something—a set of powers, an institution, or a technology—is an ethical problem when its product—an act, a system, or a technique—is capable of good or harm. The only other requirement is the mediation of human will: for the act, the system, or the technique to pose an ethical problem, it must be carried out, supervised, or participated in by persons who at some point possess, or believe themselves to possess, knowledge of their actions and the freedom to carry them out. Accidents of nature do not pose ethical problems, even if they cause harm, because they are not under human control. Should they come under such control, for example, through the creation of a technology such as amniocentesis or accurate earthquake prediction, then what was once an accident becomes, through human mediation, preventable or predictable; what was once ethically neutral becomes ethically charged. If human intervention in some form can, through its exercise or restraint, result in good or harm, then that intervention is, by its very nature, an ethical problem.

In psychiatry, powers, institutions, and technologies exist whose associated acts, systems, and techniques have the potential for good as well as harm. And, as the profession's practitioners, psychiatrists believe themselves to both know their field and have the freedom to act within it. Clearly, the field, as well as those who work in it, satisfy the criteria for ethical concern.

*Reprinted from *Psychiatric Ethics* (1981): 61–88, edited by Sidney Bloch and Paul Chodoff and used by permission of Oxford University Press, England.

Ever since psychiatry emerged as a separate discipline, it has been criticized for ethical abuses in every sphere of its activity. Probably, its ability to summarily cancel a person's freedom through its power to commit has been the subject of most such criticism: psychiatrists have required it, indeed, of persons who have not even been mentally ill. Other aspects of the profession have also been found ethically lacking. Thus, psychiatric institutions have often been seen as debasing, and the techniques of electroconvulsive therapy, behavior modification, medication, psychosurgery, and even psychotherapy have raised vexing and abiding issues regarding the control of behavior.

Potential for Error and Misuse in Psychiatric Diagnosis

But, in an important sense, all of these criticisms have missed the mark or, to be more precise, not gone deep enough. For underlying all psychiatric activities—underlying all its powers, institutions, and technologies—has been one sustaining act: diagnosis. It is the prerogative to diagnose that enables the psychiatrist to commit, that delineates the populations subjected to psychiatric care, and that sets in motion the methods used for treatment. It is this prerogative, therefore, that should provoke the most fundamental, and the most serious, ethical consideration.

Of course, the ethical problem of diagnosis—assuming that diagnosis is itself, at least in theory, a valid endeavor—has to do with its susceptibility to misuse. If enough is really known about mental disorders for practitioners to be able to categorize them, and if such categorization does indeed represent a scientifically based, or at least pragmatically useful, professional activity, then the ethical concern must be the actual or potential misapplication of diagnostic categories to persons who do not warrant or require them. Such misapplication unnecessarily places those persons at risk for the harmful effects of psychiatric diagnosis. These effects include not only the loss of personal freedom and subjection to noxious psychiatric environments and treatments, but also the possibility of life-long labeling (Balint, 1957; Scheff, 1966; Levene, 1971) as well as a variety of legal and social disadvantages ranging from declarations of nonresponsibility in family and financial affairs to, under the most extreme circumstances, the deprivation of life (Muller-Hege-mann, 1968).

In general, misdiagnoses can be said to originate in two ways. In the first way, the psychiatrist knowingly and inappropriately makes a standard psychiatric diagnosis to achieve some end that is not necessarily desired by the patient or, by common definition, medical. That end may vary. For example, the psychiatrist may be under direct and obvious pressure from a family to hospitalize a troublesome relative, or from political authorities to hospitalize a troublesome dissident. In the other way, the psychiatrist may misdiagnose at the person's own request. For example, psychiatric hospitalization may protect against a worse fate: jail, in the case of a criminal offender; the military draft, in the case of a war resister; the birth of an unwanted child, in the case of a woman seeking an abortion where it is available only to those who can show medical need. Whether or not the misdiagnosis is wanted by the diagnosee, harm results, either to the person or to the integrity of the profession.

One's main concern should certainly be for harm to the person, but harm to the profession, largely overlooked as a sort of victimless crime, also requires attention. Misdiagnoses that result from nonpurposeful causes deserve the greatest scrutiny because most misdiagnoses belong in this category. Also, misdiagnoses of the first type are, in general, clear and recognized to be unethical, while the others are more subtle and insidious, more a part of the fabric of the field itself, and much more difficult to identify and stop.

To be sure, there is a sense in which it could be argued that the second category of misdiagnoses does not constitute a true ethical problem: after all, if the misdiagnoses are not purposeful, then they do not involve knowledge or free will on the part of the psychiatrist and are beyond his or her control. But that is not quite the case. The mere fact that something is not completely purposeful does not mean that it is completely nonpurposeful. This so-called nonpurposeful category involves, in the main, nonmedical needs, pressures, and compromises that affect the diagnostic process but only partially enter the psychiatrist's awareness. The fact that the psychiatrist may, for reasons of self-comfort, ignore this awareness or a professional responsibility to strengthen it, raises this category of misdiagnoses to the highest level of ethical concern.

Nonpurposeful misdiagnoses can be traced to at least three sources, and it will be to these sources that the remainder of this discussion will be devoted.

Inherent Limitations of the Diagnostic Process

Certainly, the simplest source of misdiagnoses is the vulnerability of the diagnostic process to error. Over the years, it has been shown that the process can have a poor or questionable reliability (Mehlman, 1952; Cantwell et al., 1979; Overall & Hollister, 1979); may be subject to inconsistency and change (Babigian et al., 1965); often suffers from bias (Pasamanick et al., 1959; Babigian et al., 1965; Katz et al., 1969; Temerlin, 1970; Plutchik et al., 1972); tends to rely on subjective criteria, such as (with regard to schizophrenia) "understandability" (Jaspers, 1910; Fish, 1962; Astrup & Odegard, 1970), "peculiar behavior" (Langfeldt, 1960), "the feel of the case" (Zigler & Phillips, 1961), the "praecox feeling" (Rumke, 1950), and "bizarre thinking" (Astrachan, et al., 1972); and tends to result in diagnoses of health rather than illness because, as Scheff observed, physicians as a group feel that a "type 2 error"—accepting a hypothesis that is false—is less dangerous than a "type 1 error"—rejecting a hypothesis that is true (Scheff, 1966).

All these inherent limitations have been well described in the psychiatric literature and raise ethical questions only to the degree that they are ignored. In the absence of objective physical criteria, psychiatric diagnosis is, even in its most informed expression, only a finely tuned and intelligent art; it is the responsibility of the diagnosing psychiatrist to remember its limitations with humility and to maintain a willingness to review decisions and admit fallibility. At best, the psychiatrist is no better than his tools and must acknowledge their limitations as only the starting points of his own.

The Power of Diagnostic Theory to Shape Psychiatric Vision

But vulnerable as the diagnostic process in psychiatry is to its own limitations, limitations that may lead to misdiagnosis, and hard as the psychiatrist must try to guard against them, psychiatric diagnosis has yet other vulnerabilities, more subtle, more pervasive, more difficult to recognize, and therefore demanding even greater vigilance. Again, the danger is misdiagnosis—nonpurposeful but still damaging—and the ethical problem is the degree to which the psychiatrist may ignore the forces and circumstances that lead to, and make use of, such misdiagnosis.

In the main, diagnosis is a social act. It takes place in a social context. The psychiatrist observes behavior and judges it against a social—often local—norm. Nor is this necessarily inappropriate. Psychiatric illnesses, particularly those characterized by psychosis, often affect persons in ways that lead them to violate social norms and to traverse generally accepted verbal and behavioral boundaries; such trespasses may, in fact, be the most sensitive and early indicators of illness. To be sure, the social basis of diagnosis is itself a problem, since the psychiatrist must judge precisely where the social boundaries should be drawn and which trespasses are the result not of illness but of some other cause, for example, social activism, artistic style, mere eccentricity, or, for that matter, a rearing in another culture. But most psychiatrists are aware of these problems, at least dimly, having been apprised of them during training or, failing that, in the course of ongoing practice.

However, another basis for diagnostic judgment—one that shapes the diagnostic vision of the psychiatrist no less powerfully than social considerations but is, nevertheless, generally unrecognized—is diagnostic theory itself. In most countries, psychiatrists are guided by one or more theories of mental illness, often associated with diagnostic systems that are the functional and practical expressions of the theories. And, depending on the specificity of the adopted system, the way the psychiatrist assesses a person's behavior, draws conclusions about it, weighs the variance between the behavior and the social norm—indeed, *sees* the person—may be heavily influenced by the assumptions underlying the system and the approach that system takes to recognize and identify mental illness. The system, after all, delineates categories of illness and identifies the criteria by which behaviors and the persons who exhibit them are placed in those categories. Also, every time such a placement is made, the categories, as well as the system itself, are reified. To the psychiatrist who accepts the system as real, this occasions no concern: the reality of the system has merely found a correspondence in the reality of the patient's illness.

However, to one who finds the categories mistaken, or the criteria too narrowly or too broadly defined, such reification may simply be self-deceiving and false, and may result in misdiagnoses as systematic as only a system can cause.

In many countries, this danger is relatively small. The competition of theories is so great and the impact of systems so circumscribed or diluted that, while errors may result, their scale is necessarily limited. In the United States at this time, for example, contrasting theories—such as those stressing psychological causation and those stressing the biological basis of mental illness—actively compete to such an extent without official sanction or encouragement from governmental or professional bodies that the diagnostic system in use, even if it is itself codified and official, can hardly represent a unified approach to mental illness. Thus, the system is unlikely to impose on the psychiatrist a rigid vision of psychiatric reality to be adopted as the basis for a strict model of the psychiatrist's own sense of the nature, meaning, and limits of psychopathology.

In some countries, however—one, at least—the danger of such an imposition is not only great but, indeed, the imposition is already evident. In that country, psychiatrists have adopted an understanding of mental illness based on the theoretical teachings of a dominant school; have accepted, whole, an approach to diagnosis in accordance with the rules of that school's formal and elaborate system; and have come to see—really see—persons as naturally and precisely falling into the categories that make up that system. That country is the Soviet Union, and its experience has much to teach about the ways in which an official diagnostic system can shape psychiatric vision and skew diagnostic practice, ensnaring persons who elsewhere would be considered mentally well in the broad net that defines them, irrevocably, as mentally ill. The Soviet experience is important because it exemplifies, in pure and extreme form, a trend only now developing in other countries, including the United States; because its effects can be documented in multiple ways; and because it demonstrates, with grim clarity, how a system that appears to have only scientific origins and professional goals can, simply by virtue of its own nature as a systematic psychiatric technology, result in significant human harm.

What has happened in the Soviet Union has been the development during the past two decades of a diagnostic system that is by now standard in Moscow and nearly so in the rest of the country. The system was developed during the 1960s by Andrei V. Snezhnevsky, the founder of what has come to be called the Moscow School of psychiatry and the head of the Institute of Psychiatry of the U.S.S.R. Academy of Medical Sciences, the central psychiatric research center in that country. During the 1940s and 1950s, Snezhnevsky worked at and then became chairman of the Department of Psychiatry of the Central Postgraduate Medical Institute, to which the most talented academic psychiatrists in the country came to obtain their advanced degrees. Upon his ascension to the directorship of the Institute of Psychiatry in 1962, he dedicated the Institute and its resources to the problem of schizophrenia, which was the focus of his central theory and diagnostic approach. Over the next decade, he and his staff continued to refine the system, doing clinical research designed to elaborate its details. By the early 1970s, many of his former students and trainees were in charge of the nation's academic psychiatric centers; the journal he edited, the *Korsakov Journal of Neuropathology and Psychiatry*, was the only psychiatric periodical in the U.S.S.R. and regularly carried news of his school's research and of the fine points of its diagnostic system; and the pattern of psychiatric teaching and research in centers far from Moscow felt the effect of his guidance and views, exerted through his role as an influential member of review committees for government ministries responsible for the approval of research and training grants. By the middle and late 1970s, the hegemony of the Moscow School was almost complete: it was, clearly, the dominant force in Soviet psychiatry, and its system the standard Soviet approach to mental illness.

The system itself focuses on schizophrenia but, because its definition of schizophrenia is so extraordinarily broad, takes in vast sectors of psychopathology which, grouped together, encompass almost the whole of mental illness.

The theory behind the system is based on the assumption that schizophrenia has three different forms; that these forms vary from each other not so much in their symptoms, as traditionally assumed in the West since Kraepelin, but in their course; and that the form represented by a particular schizophrenic's course may be identified on the basis of a retrospective analysis of the development of his or her illness (Snezhnevsky & Vartanyan, 1970; Snezhnevsky, 1971a, b; Nadzharov, 1972).

A schematic rendering of the features of the three course forms is presented in figure 1. The continuous form is characterized by the development of symptoms early in life, usually by late adolescence or early adulthood, with a general worsening as life progresses. Patients falling into this category do not, as a rule, improve. The periodic form is characterized by periods of acute illness interspersed with periods of remission during which health is regained. The shift-like form is a mixture of the other two; there are periodic acute attacks, but each attack leaves the patient more ill than before so that, overall, there is a continuing general worsening of the illness during the course of the patient's life.

What is so unique—and, in the end, so problematic—about this system is the fact that two of the course forms, the continuous and the shift-like, have subtypes ranging from mild to severe, and that the mild subtypes are characterized by symptoms that are not psychotic. In almost all countries, psychiatrists would probably agree, by their own criteria, that persons who satisfy the Moscow School's criteria for moderate and severe subtypes really are schizophrenic. But they would probably disagree with the Moscow School's criteria for mild subtypes and judge such persons to be neurotic, not schizophrenic, suffering from a character disorder, or even mentally well.

The other feature of the system that adds to its potential danger—indeed, multiplies it—is the assumption, developed over the past decade, that each of the course forms represents, in essence, a separate illness, one that has its own biological basis, which is, in turn, genetically determined. This implies that a person placed in, say, the sluggish (mild) subtype of the continuous form has the same illness as anyone else in that form, including someone in the malignant (severe) subtype, and, though the person has a more mildly expressed version of that illness, the illness is present—and persists for life. Such a person may therefore be subject to many of the same disadvantages, social and personal, as those much more severely ill.

What is so troubling about this is clearly that the criteria given for mild subtypes of schizophrenia apply to many persons who would be seen by most psychiatrists as not schizophrenic at all. In fact, it could be predicted that, applied to a broad population, this system would draw into the schizophrenic fold precisely such persons who have neuroses, character disorders, affective

COURSE FORMS						
Continuous			**Periodic**	**Shift-Like**		
LIFE COURSE OF THE ILLNESS 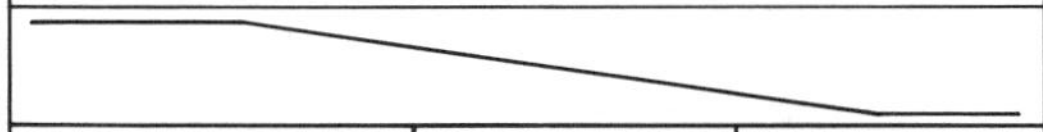 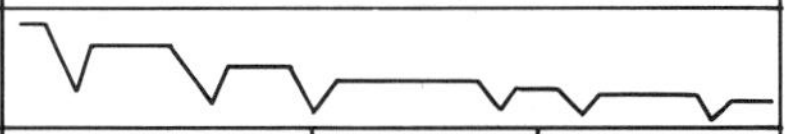 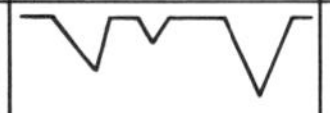						
Sluggish (Mild)	*Paranoid (Moderate)*	*Malignant (Severe)*		*Mild*	*Moderate*	*Severe*
Neurotic; self-consciousness; introspectiveness; obsessive doubts; conflicts with parental and other authorities; "reformism"	Paranoid; delusions; hallucinations; "parasitic life style"	Early onset; unremitting; overwhelming	Acute attacks; fluctuations in mood; confusion	Neurotic, with affective coloring; social conten-tiousness; philosophical concerns; self-absorption	Acute paranoid	Catatonia; delusions; prominent mood changes

Row labels (left margin): LIFE COURSE OF THE ILLNESS; SUBTYPES; SOME CHARACTERISTICS

FIGURE 1

Features of the Snezhnevsky Course Forms

illnesses, and no mental illnesses at all. And, in fact, there is evidence that this has occurred.

Some of the evidence is impressionistic. Rollins, for example, reported in her book on child psychiatry in the Soviet Union that patients with primarily neurotic or psychopathic-like symptoms were typically given diagnoses by Soviet psychiatrists in the schizophrenic range (Rollins, 1972). More directly, Holland reported, after a sojourn in Moscow's Institute of Psychiatry, that Soviet patients may be diagnosed as schizophrenic even if they exhibit no signs of the illness, and that, once the diagnosis is given, even if further subtyped as mild, it continues to be used on the assumption that the patient has a life-long, genetically based condition (Hite, 1974; Holland & Shakhmatova-Pavolva, 1974; Holland, 1975; Holland, 1977a, b).

But the most telling evidence has come from the International Pilot Study of Schizophrenia (IPSS), carried out during the late 1960s and early 1970s in nine centers around the world, including Washington and Moscow, which evaluated patients for schizophrenia and collected data about them. The center in Moscow was Snezhnevsky's Institute of Psychiatry. As part of the study, a computer was programmed by John K. Wing to rediagnose patients originally diagnosed as schizophrenic at the various centers, using data regarding the patients' symptoms that were gathered by the center itself; the computer used strict criteria for its own rediagnoses, notably those formulated by Kurt Schneider (WHO, 1973). While most centers did "well"—that is, the computer "agreed" with most diagnoses of schizophrenia rendered at those centers—two centers did poorly.

One of these two, Washington, did poorly, it turns out, primarily because its diagnosticians followed the rules of their own diagnostic system and, unlike the computer, tended not to differentiate between schizophrenia, schizophrenia-like psychoses, and paranoid psychoses; the computer gave them low marks only because it found their schizophrenics to be, by its criteria, otherwise psychotic. The agreement as to the presence of psychosis, however, was high.

The other center that did poorly in computer rediagnoses was Moscow's Institute of Psychiatry, but in that case the reasons were different. A larger percentage of Moscow's diagnosed schizophrenics were reassigned by the computer not to psychotic but to depressive and neurotic categories. Table 1 shows

TABLE 1
Computer Classifications of Schizophrenia Subtype Diagnoses for International Pilot Study of Schizophrenia (IPSS)

IPSS Center	Schizophrenia Subtype Diagnoses	No. of Patients	Computer Classifications, %				
			Schizophrenic & Similar Psychoses	Paranoid Psychoses	Manic Psychoses	Depressive Psychoses	Depressive Neuroses
Washington	Simple	4	50	33	17	0	0
	Latent	2					
Moscow	Sluggish	12	0	0	33	8	58
Seven Remaining Centers	Simple	27	71	9	6	0	14
	Latent	8					

the computer classification (i.e., rediagnosis) of patients originally diagnosed at the nine centers as belonging to subtypes most likely to contain patients who would be considered by psychiatrists in many countries to be "borderline schizophrenics" or merely "borderline," that is, mildly ill and possibly not psychotic. For eight of the centers, these subtypes were identified as "simple" and "latent." For Moscow, it was "sluggish" (the mild subtype of the Moscow School's continuous form). Although the numbers were small, the difference seems striking. Patients placed in these subtypes at eight of the centers, including Washington but not Moscow, were classified by the computer as overwhelmingly schizophrenic or as having paranoid or schizophrenia-like psychoses. Patients placed in the mild subtype by the Moscow diagnosticians, following the rules of the Moscow School, were classified by the computer as primarily affectively ill or depressed, just as one might have predicted from an inspection of the system's broad diagnostic criteria (Reich, 1975).

Finally, another confirmation of the tendency of the Moscow School's diagnostic system to overdiagnose schizophrenia has come from a Soviet psychiatrist working at Moscow's Serbsky Institute of Forensic Psychiatry. In an unprecedented article in a Western psychiatric journal, E. P. Kazanetz used his own computer exercise to show that the Moscow School's system tended to overdiagnose as endogenous schizophrenics persons who were only exogenously ill—that is, it tended to diagnose as chronically ill persons whose illnesses were primarily of an acute, externally caused type. Furthermore, Kazanetz added the observation that such overdiagnosis could be harmful to persons with acute illnesses assigned irrevocably to psychiatric registers of the chronically ill. Together with the evidence from the IPSS, Kazanetz's study reveals the degree to which an overly broad diagnostic scheme can result in overly broad diagnostic practice (Reich, 1979a, b).

What is so extraordinary about the Soviet experience, and ethically so significant, is that the patients in the IPSS and in the population studied by Kazanetz who were misdiagnosed as schizophrenic—despite the fact that almost all other psychiatrists would diagnose them as belonging in less severe categories of mental illness—were misdiagnosed only because of the dictates of the official diagnostic system. These Soviet psychiatrists really *saw* the patients as schizophrenic; or, to put it another way, *the system created a category, first on paper and then, with training, in the minds of Sovet psychiatrists, that was eventually assumed to represent a real class of patients and was inevitably filled by real persons.* Those diagnosticians came to see schizophrenic pathology as including very mild forms and diagnosed accordingly. Persons who should not have received such diagnoses did, to their detriment; and psychiatrists who should not have given such diagnoses did, in apparent good faith. Had those psychiatrists been sensitive to the capacity of diagnostic systems to shape the way psychiatrists understand, categorize, and perceive psychopathology, they might have been able, one hopes, to avert this result.

Nor should the Soviet experience be seen as exotic or unique. The Soviet diagnostic scheme represents an extreme spectrum system that posits a spectrum of schizophrenic illness ranging in severity from the most mild to the most severe and caused by a genetic deficit of variable clinical expression. Such diagnostic schemes are, in fact, under active consideration in the West (Rosenthal, 1963; Kety et al., 1968, 1975, 1978a, b; Rosenthal et al., 1968, 1971; Wender et al., 1974; Fowler et al., 1975; Reich, 1976a, b; Rieder, 1978). To be sure, these schemes remain only under examination and have not yet been introduced into formal diagnostic systems. However, given the Soviet experience, it would be valuable to weigh the potential of such systems for similar overdiagnoses; not to do so at this point may constitute a kind of ethical trespass.

The Beauty of Diagnosis as a Solution to Human Problems

A third, and probably most significant, source of nonpurposeful psychiatric misdiagnoses is the attractiveness of the diagnostic process as a means of solving or avoiding complex human problems. With remarkable ease, diagnoses can turn the fright of chaos into the comfort of the known, the burden of doubt into the pleasure of certainty, the shame of hurting others into the pride of helping them, and the dilemma of moral judgment into the opaque clarity of medical truth. Because of their nature, functions, and meanings, diagnoses can do such things in efficient and powerful ways and make their use by psychiatrists for such ends remarkably irresistible, enormously unrecognizable, and, in the final analysis, utterly and failingly human (Reich, 1980).

Diagnosis as Explanation, Mitigation, and Exculpation. Perhaps the most fetching beauty of diagnosis is its capacity to instantly explain: odd, objectionable, troublesome, or illegal behavior can be, through the mediation of diagnosis, suddenly understood, explained, and explained away. To be sure, such behavior may indeed be the product of diagnosable mental illness, but the capacity of diagnosis to provide instant explanation makes its use tempting even in cases in which such illness does not exist or is, at best, only marginally present.

The arena in which this diagnostic temptation has been most evident is the law. For years, psychiatrists have been asked to testify as witnesses in cases of persons accused of various crimes. Often, both the prosecution and the defense have called upon such witnesses, who, in turn, have presented conflicting testimony about whether the actions carried out by the accused were a product of mental illness. While such conflicts have occasionally embarrassed the profession by suggesting that either side can get psychiatric testimony to support any desired diagnosis, at least they have been straightforward. Generally, the clinical questions have had to do with the presence or absence of some kind of psychosis, a group of mental conditions that can render a defendant legally not responsible for the actions in question; and the testimony has usually involved judgments about whether or not the defendant's behavior and history met certain widely accepted criteria for these most agreed-upon areas of psychopathology. Naturally, defendants and defense counsels have often sought findings of "not guilty by reason of insanity," even when they suspected or knew that insanity had not played a role, because they believed that, at least for such serious crimes as murder or rape, hospital confinement was preferable to the sentence likely to be imposed should the defendant be found guilty and not insane. Still, some persons *do* commit crimes because they are insane, and the law recognizes that insanity compromises free will and classifies someone without free will as legally not responsible for his or her actions. Defendants have the right to use that defense, and psychiatrists have a role, as a result of their expertise in recognizing such mental illness, in testifying on the substance of that defense.

The trouble is that, in recent years, attempts have been made to expand that role into realms in which psychiatrists do not have expertise, deriving from the wish to have diagnostically explained—and legally explained away—criminal behaviors that do not involve classical psychotic states. Instead of insanity, many clinical questions have involved issues, primarily of coercion, persusasion, and influence, about which psychiatry has almost no validated knowledge. In a series of cases, defense attorneys have turned to psychiatrists to testify about the effects of certain environmental pressures on individual development and judgment, and on the role these factors played in the genesis of the criminal behavior. The defense argument has usually been that these factors created a diagnosable mental condition that explained the behavior and, in a legal sense, either mitigated or totally exculpated it.

The best-known case of this sort was the 1976 bank robbery trial of Patricia Hearst, in which the defendant was said to have been incapable of criminal intent because she had undergone a process of "coercive persuasion," which had affected her capacity for free will. In a sense, not only the defense, but also many observers, favored such a diagnostic exculpation because it made it possible to understand how such an ordinary, peaceful, apolitical, and utterly American young woman could have turned so suddenly into such an extraordinary, violent, ideological, and anti-American revolutionary. The court allowed that novel defense—novel because it stepped beyond the traditional realm of insanity into the broader arena of persuasion—and a battery of psychiatrists supported it with their testimony. The jury, however, rejected it, despite its attractive advantages. Diagnostic explanation, they found, was not, at least in their eyes, a basis for legal exculpation (Reich, 1976a, b).

The attractiveness of the diagnostic process as a means of explanation and exculpation has revealed itself in the legal arena several times since the Hearst trial. In each instance, the defense contended that environmental factors had influenced or determined the criminal act; and, in each instance, psychiatrists took the stand with supporting diagnostic opinions. In one celebrated Florida case, for example, a young boy accused of having killed an old woman was defended with the explanation that his mind had been affected by television violence. As in the Hearst trial, the jury found such use of diagnosis inadequate to explain away the defendant's behavior.

Despite these setbacks, it seems likely that the beauty of diagnosis will continue to be appreciated in the legal arena, and that psychiatrists will continue to expand the ambit of their diagnostic expertise into areas about which almost nothing certain is known. It seems possible that psychiatric testimony will in time offer itself in support of psychosocial defenses of all kinds, for example, the attribution of criminal actions to the defendant's early childhood rearing or to the pressures of adolescent peers. While such influences undoubtedly exist, almost nothing is known about how they affect the capacity for individual judgment and the exercise of free will. That psychiatrists are willing to testify on these matters in the belief that they have such knowledge demonstrates not only the settled habit of psychiatrists to opine on issues beyond their scientific domain but also, it seems, the satisfaction gained from finding in the storehouse of the profession some explanation that will transform a person's criminal act into a symptom, a painful moral question into a painless medical finding.

Nor should the turn of psychiatrists to diagnosis in such cases occasion any wonder. It is a natural turn when an explanation for unwanted behavior is needed and is performed every day outside the courts by nonpsychiatric laymen as well. For example, journalists and other observers turn to it for simplifying explanations when political figures engage in behavior that is inexplicable in ordinary political terms (Evans & Novak, 1979; Gup, 1979; Quinn, 1979; Schram, 1979; Sinclair, 1979; *Washington Post*, 1979). Still others call upon diagnostic explanations to justify forgiveness or elicit sympathy in situations ranging from breaches of airline etiquette (*Newsweek*, 1979) to more serious transgressions of industry ethics (Berry & Egan, 1977) and literary propriety (Mitgang, 1979). That psychiatrists similarly turn to diagnoses in the search for satisfying explanatory simplification, which substitute medicine for morals, is therefore not surprising; the satisfactions and advantages are the same except that psychiatric diagnoses achieve official status and recognition and result in lasting effects that are not always, even in these cases, salutary.

Diagnosis as Reassurance. A second beauty of diagnosis is its power to reassure. When acts are committed whose implications are disturbing—acts that suggest vulnerabilities in ourselves, our institutions, or our communal beliefs—diagnoses often come to mind, both in the layman and in the psychiatrist, that serve to shift the frame of the behavior from the threatening personal or social arena to a safer medical one.

In one widely publicized case, for example, this shift was effected toward its reassuring end through the cooperation of all concerned, psychiatrist and laymen alike. In 1974, Dr. William T. Summerlin, a young researcher hired by the Memorial–Sloan Kettering Cancer Center on the basis of his promising work in transplantation immunology, reported that he had successfully grafted skin with genetically unrelated animals. When other researchers were unable to confirm these astonishing results, Summerlin repeated his experiments and inked in the skins of his mice to make it appear that the grafts had taken.

When this scientific fraud was revealed by Summerlin's research assistant, a special in-house committee was constituted to investigate the matter. The major threat posed by the Summerlin affair was the possibility that the American public might conclude that not only that researcher, but research itself, was suspect. To a research community that depended on the magnificent largesse of its various constituents and supporters—at that time over two billion dollars a year from U.S. government sources alone—such a prospect was indeed distressing. Moreover, there were other concerns. Summerlin's story, after all, did violence to the new American dream—a young man from the country's heartland, embraced by the eastern scientific establishment, proves himself shamefully unreliable. What of that dream? And, besides, what was to become of young Summerlin himself?

The solution to these distressing concerns was quick in coming. First, the investigating committee issued its findings: Summerlin's "unusual behavior involved at least a measure of self-deception, or some other aberration, which hindered him from adequately gauging the impact and eventual results of his conduct" (Brody, 1974a). Then, at a press conference, the cancer center's president, Dr. Lewis Thomas, a researcher and physician himself, informed the assembled reporters, "The fraud in this work was a result of mental illness" (Brody, 1974b).

In one stroke, all concerns were eased. Summerlin's actions were the result not of a vulnerability in research or the habits of researchers, but, rather, of a fault in the man. Moreover, that fault was not moral, but medical. And besides that, it was short-lived. At his own news conference, four days later, Summerlin offered that he had been suffering from an acute depression which accounted for his "irrational act" and for which he had already begun psychiatric treatment. The psychiatrist, Summerlin explained, had prescribed rest and physical exercise, and he was already feeling much better. And so, indeed, did those who had been so distressed by the implications of Summerlin's act. The diagnosis preserved not only the good name of science and the integrity of the scientific community but also Summerlin, who could be seen now, in more reassuring terms, not as a person who would be forever morally tainted but as one whose treatment would leave him clean, whole, and good, ready to resume his professional life.

Whether Summerlin's behavior was or was not, in fact, the result of an acute depression cannot, of course, be confirmed here, but the case is important because it illustrates the ease with which a turn to diagnosis can, at the same time, allay multiple concerns. When a psychiatrist is faced by such a case, when an available means—the diagnostic process—can accomplish so much, and when others are themselves inclined to think that mental illness can or should be used to explain the behavior, then it is hard to imagine that the psychiatrist will not look seriously at that option, even consider it with greater favor than might be the case with similar behaviors that posed no threat or raised no concerns.

Diagnosis as the Humane Transformation of Social Deviance into Medical Illness. Another beauty of diagnosis is its power to reclassify whole categories of socially unacceptable behavior as the products of psychiatrically diagnosable conditions. This kind of reclassification derives, in essence, from a liberal utopian impulse: people are naturally good, and someone who acts to the detriment of society must be ill. Hence, the social response should aim not at punishment, or mere control, but at treatment. If this approach is taken, everyone presumably benefits: the deviant, the "root causes" of whose transgressions are thereby recognized and cured; society and its authorities, which are no longer in the position of exacting harsh punishments; and psychiatrists, whose redefinitions make all this possible and who can feel themselves in the noble position of healing where others would have only hurt.

Probably the most striking examples of such reclassifications may be found in connection with sexual behaviors traditionally considered socially undesirable. As a result of developments in medical technology, as well as shifts in popular views, some of these behaviors have been reclassified in psychiatric—and, therefore, diagnostic—terms. One such development, the synthesis of drugs that reduce sexual drive, has resulted in calls for their use on sexual offenders. One drug company, for example, advertised in the *British Journal of Psychiatry* that its product "has proven to be of value in treating men who have been guilty of sexual offenses such as exhibitionism; paedophilia; indecent assault; rape; incest; voyeurism; bestiality and paederasty." The company also pointed out that other types of "aberrant" sexual behaviors, even those not considered illegal, may also be "controlled," including "homosexual activities; fetishism; transvestism; compulsive masturbation; and sexual aggression in senile or mentally defective hospital patients." In the United States, prisoners serving jail sentences for rape have gone to court demanding that they be treated with similar agents (Colen, 1975). Developments of a surgical type have made still other "treatment" options available, with individuals and their doctors rushing in to reclassify the aberrancy or malady in medical terms tailored to fit the new treatments—and the increasing demands.

The danger here is that, despite their humanitarian goal, such reclassifications may not be serving that end. Attributing to an exhibitionist, a rapist, or a voyeur an underlying diagnosable psychiatric condition—hypersexualism—and then treating that condition by pharmacological or surgical means are not necessarily humane, and, in fact, not yet proven to work. Indeed, the surgical approach to transsexuality, a darling of 1960s medical technology, has only recently been shown to be seriously questionable (Myer & Reter, 1979). Certainly, it is not at all clear that such redefinitions have improved the lots of the persons redefined.

Analogous reclassifications have also been attempted in other areas of psychiatry, with equally questionable results for both the professionals and their newly classified patients. Young offenders, for example, have been told by courts and other authorities that they would not be punished for their drug-taking or other social trespasses if they submitted to psychiatric treatment; and psychiatrists and psychiatric hospitals sometimes have acquiesced in this process by making their practices, facilities, and diagnoses available to these offenders, usually in good faith and full belief. Instead of being recorded as criminals, such persons have been hospitalized as sociopaths or, sometimes, latent or mild schizophrenics. The labels and consequent treatment have had inadvertently worse effects on the individuals than would have resulted from an original designation as deviants or criminals.

Diagnosis as Exclusion and Dehumanization. The discussion so far has examined the beauty of diagnosis as a means of accomplishing ends that in some sense reflect the universal wish to be or do good. From time to time, we all have an urge to exculpate, to reassure, and to turn deviance into illness; diagnosis does these things, does them magically and utterly, and, in resorting to diagnosis, both laymen and psychiatrists have what they think are the diagnosee's interest at heart.

But the diagnostic process has a beauty that leads well beyond the realm of generous human interest. We also use it because it helps us do things we otherwise could not bring ourselves to do.

The roots of such use are primitive, powerful, and universal. When we want to do unto others as we would not have them do unto us, we find some way of turning them into "others" who are not "us." We usually do that by labeling them, excluding them from our own group, and dehumanizing them by defining their status as less than ours and, therefore, less human.

Stalin knew that, and did it on a national scale when he wanted to turn popular opinion against those who disagreed with him. Khrushchev, in his 1956 Twentieth Party Congress speech, described the process well. Stalin, he said:

originated the concept of "enemy of the people." This term automatically rendered it unnecessary that the ideological errors of a man or men engaged in a controversy be proven; this term made possible the usage of the most cruel repression, violating all norms of revolutionary legality, against anyone who in any way disagreed with Stalin. . . (Khrushchev, 1970, p. 566).

Stalin understood that a person labeled "an enemy of the people" would be seen by a wary and besieged population as a dangerous outsider who must be excluded from Soviet society. So seen, the outsider would be suddenly transformed into someone who is different, not truly a member of society, not truly a man—someone who therefore could and should be imprisoned, shot, or otherwise silenced without the sympathy ordinarily accorded a nonlabeled fellow comrade.

In her remarkable memoir of her life with Osip Mandelstam, *Hope Against Hope*, Nadezhda Mandelstam, the poet's widow, located in Lenin himself the origin of the Soviet tendency to distinguish between "one of us" and "not one of us" (the second group commonly being known as "alien elements"). Lenin, she pointed out, established that distinction during the Civil War with his "Who whom," the phrase he used to summarize the difference between the Bolsheviks and their enemies (Mandelstam, 1970, p. 28). She also showed how widespread was the tendency under Stalin, even among the intelligentsia, to exclude and dehumanize those officially cast out. Thus, when an acquaintance was arrested on unknown and usually arbitrary charges, people told each other—probably to reassure themselves that they would not be next—that "he isn't one of us." It was, for many, necessary "to avoid those stricken by the plague" (Mandelstam, 1970, p. 26).

Even more graphic examples of the dehumanizing power of labeling, and the universal tendency to use it, can be drawn from the context of war. In World War II, both sides had ways of turning each other into objects whose deaths would be less than tragic, somehow almost deserved. The Nazis pushed this stratagem to its limits, using labeling to transform Jews, Gypsies, homosexuals, and sometimes Slavs into vermin whose extermination would be a blessing and should certainly occasion no discomfort in the heart of a good Aryan.

And even in Vietnam the martial advantages of labeling, exclusion, and dehumanization revealed themselves. American soldiers were given the task there of fighting an enemy often indistinguishable from the general population. Any Vietnamese man, woman, or child was potentially lethal, so all became the enemy, and one had to be ready to kill them. In order to be able to do that, one had to see them as not being in the same class as onself. One called them "dinks" and "gooks"; one saw them as "nothing but whores or thieves" (Lifton, 1973, p. 194). Many an American soldier thus transformed the Vietnamese population into objects he could annihilate without the danger of annihilating himself through guilt. The power of this process was illustrated by a soldier who had to move corpses found after a battle. American corpses were bodies, while Vietnamese corpses felt, to him, like "potato sacks." In carrying them, he told an interviewing psychiatrist, Robert Jay Lifton, he "didn't feel a thing" (Lifton, 1973, p. 192).

Diagnosis is perfectly suited to label, exclude, and dehumanize in both its informal and formal usages. Informally, the terms "crazy," "mad," and even "schizophrenic" often serve as exclusionary labels in everyday language to identify others who are annoying, discomfiting, and different. Formally applied—that is, by psychiatrists—a diagnosis can make a person into someone who seems wholly other and who *requires* exclusion, someone who, depending on the severity of the diagnosis, may be seen by others as disordered, polluted, and dangerous. In short, a diagnosis can convert a person into another kind of human being, perhaps less than human, certainly not a fellow human being, who not only must but deserves to be put away. Such diagnostic transformation can serve the needs of psychiatric systems under certain conditions in exactly the same way that it can serve the needs of family and social systems when their peace and tranquillity are disturbed by the symptoms of the mentally ill.

Psychiatric systems may need the process of diagnostic exclusion and dehumanization to be able to subject individuals to treatment experiences and conditions difficult to impose without such preparatory diagnostic transformation. Psychiatric hospitals, especially of the public variety, may be unpleasant places, and some psychiatric techniques, such as the use of drugs, electric shock, restraints, and confinement to seclusion rooms, may be experienced by patients as highly noxious. The psychiatrist knows that hospitalization in the service of treatment may also cause a patient a certain degree of harm. The awareness of possible harm is compounded if the patient does not seek treatment voluntarily, if the most invasive or liberty-depriving techniques are used, and if the patient resists with denials of sickness and pleas for alteration or cessation of treatment and immediate release.

At such times, the psychiatrist must harden his or her heart. What makes this possible is, among other things, the diagnosis. With it, the person is seen as a patient, whose pleas are not simple, soulful, human importunings but routine and expected reactions to distressing illness and perturbing treatment. With the diagnosis, the psychiatrist can proceed, feeling not like a violator of human freedom and dignity but like a healer helping, through hospitalization and therapeutic interventions, to transform a psychiatric case back into a human being, back into someone like the psychiatrist. As a psychiatrist, one can thus, in good conscience, allow oneself to do unto the patient that which one would not have others do unto oneself.

The advantage to the psychiatrist of diagnostic dehumanization is only a special instance of that advantage in everyday life. After all, psychiatric patients carry on the largest portions of their lives outside the psychiatric system and confront nonpsychiatrists with similar, even more vexing, dilemmas. The behaviors of such patients may be extremely distressing to friends, neighbors, and relatives who, in turn, seek help for themselves by convincing or coercing the individual to consult mental health authorities, enlisting others, such as the police, to carry out coercion if needed. Sometimes, these friends, neighbors, or relatives may later feel shame when they recognize that their wish to be rid of the individual and their actions to accomplish that end were partly for their own comfort, especially if the patient must suffer unpleasant treatment. That shame can be dissipated by the reminder that the patient is, in fact, mentally ill, that the objectionable behaviors were caused not by the person but the disease, and that purpose of seeking help from civil and mental health authorities was related not to the needs of those feeling shame but to the needs of the person temporarily beset by a disease. The disease has obscured the patient's usual humanity and made it necessary and virtuous to do to one person what, if done to others, would represent cruelty or a transgression of civil liberties but here represents only kindness, concern, and the desire to restore an afflicted individual to the normal community of man.

Of course, persons do become psychotic and do, in their psychoses, sometimes require interventions we would not want done to ourselves. What is important here is understanding the capacity of diagnosis to enable others who respect and even love such psychotic individuals to suspend a habitual compliance with the individuals' wishes, that is, to reverse the usual meaning of compassion so that what the psychotic wants is precisely the opposite of what is given. If diagnosis can do that in such cases, then it also has a great capacity to do it in other cases that involve no respect or love. For example, if someone marginally ill annoys others by socially unacceptable behavior, it may become too easy to use an informal diagnosis as cause for, say, civil authorities to enlist the psychiatric system in both removing the disturbance and justifying the action by confirming the diagnosis. Also, it may become too easy for those in the psychiatric system to acquiesce and issue a diagnosis—even when the diagnosis may be somewhat doubtful and the consequences unpleasant—on the basis of the self-deceiving rationale that a diagnosed individual is not quite a person and probably needs treatment, at least until it takes effect, exorcises the disease, and restores a fully human state.

Diagnosis as Self-Confirming Hypothesis. Perhaps the most remarkable property of diagnosis and sometimes, for the diagnosed patient, the most enraging, is its capacity for inevitable self-confirmation. That property is evident in everyday life when people are called "crazy," "weird," or similar psychopathologizing epithets, which thereafter are used as lay diagnoses to explain or dismiss all suspect behavior. In fact, every subsequent action can become proof that the original assessment was correct.

This "catch-22" quality of pathological naming functions with even greater efficiency and inevitability within psychiatry itself, as illustrated by an actual clinical case. The chief psychiatrist at a medical school teaching hospital was asked to see a 65-year-old woman by the woman's son, a medical school faculty member, and by her husband, a physician in a nearby community. The woman, they explained, had become negative at home, disagreeable, more insistent than she previously had been about her views, and, in other ways as well, had undergone changes in personality. The chief psychiatrist, who tended to interpret behavior and its aberrations as direct products of brain functioning or malfunctioning, concluded that a malfunctioning had in fact taken place. He diagnosed an organic brain syndrome, probably caused by aging, and admitted the woman to the hospital to confirm the diagnosis.

The resident psychiatrist assigned to the case, however, could find no objective evidence of such malfunctioning. Meanwhile, the patient—finding herself in the strange circumstances of a therapeutic community in which staff and patients were expected to aid each other in recognizing illness and in promoting health—became extremely distressed. She repeatedly insisted to all who would hear and at every community or group meeting that she was not ill and should not be a patient. The response was consistent: she would certainly not have been admitted to the hospital had she not been ill, and the only way for her to achieve health was to acknowledge her illness. At first, she tried quietly to accept the ward routines in the hope that she would be discharged rapidly. When this failed, she complained loudly, angrily, and at length. The senior medical and nursing staff, observing her behavior, cited it to the resident as a "catastrophic reaction" so typical of persons with her diagnosis when challenged by tasks they can no longer master. Given fluphenazine, she quieted, and the drug-induced response was then cited as an improvement that further demonstrated the validity of the original diagnosis.

Of course, the diagnosis may indeed have been correct: the resident may have been wrong and the chief right. But, given the authority structure of the ward and the nature and effects of diagnosis, particularly those issued in such settings, it became almost inevitable that the chief's clinical pronouncement would confirm itself no matter what occurred. In the absence of objective, physically based criteria, many psychiatric diagnoses are capable of such self-confirmation, whether they derive from a psychoanalytic orientation or, as in this case, an organicist one. Indeed, even in this case, in which a psychiatric diagnosis was issued that is more susceptible to physical confirmation than most, the lack of such confirmation failed to derail the inevitable train of events. In such a climate, it becomes simply too easy to diagnose: one is rarely proved wrong, and the penchant for rapid assessment, valued so highly in general medical (especially academic) settings as an emblem of knowledge and expertise, can be exercised with few means of objective checks in the psychiatric arena, and can result in too cavalier an issuance of diagnoses. Such diagnoses, because they may be wrong, and because they have so pronounced a tendency to persist, can be highly distressing and, ultimately, damaging. Of course, this dilemma is worse under circumstances in which diagnoses reflect not academic showmanship or ideological bias but hasty or uncaring judgments. Whatever the circumstances, the results to the patient are the same.

Diagnosis as Discreditation and Punishment. And, finally, the ultimate function of diagnosis in everyday life, classical in every respect, is as universal as the species and as old as man: diagnosis as discreditation, the attribution of a person's views, politics, actions, or conclusions to a mind gone sick—diagnosis as a weapon.

We see it everywhere. In the Middle East, for example, the Shah, before losing power, identified Libya's Colonel Qadaffi as a "crazy fellow" (*New York Times*, 1976). In turn, Ahmed Zaki Yamani, the Saudi oil minister, described the Shah as "highly unstable mentally" (Anderson & Whitten, 1976). Egypt's President Sadat diagnosed Ayatollah Ruhollah Khomeini as "a lunatic" (*New York Times*, 1979), a compliment the Ayatollah passed on to President Carter (Anderson & Whitten, 1976). In Israel, the Labor opposition had similar views about Prime Minister Begin (Farrell, 1978) while, on the West Bank, Ali Jabari, the Palestinian mayor of Hebron, campaigned to have the leaders of the Palestine Liberation Organization (PLO) locked up in insane asylums (Randal, 1979).

And elsewhere, too, and at other times. Thus Lenin, in 1919, to Gorky: ". . . all of your impressions are totally sick . . . your nerves have obviously broken down. . . . Just as your conversation, your letter is the sum total of sick impressions carrying you to sick conclusions. This is all a pure sick psyche. . . . It is clear that you have worked yourself up into sickness. . . ." (Lenin, 1975). The Soviet press on the dissident physicist Sakharov: "pathological individualism" (*Washington Post*, 1977). A West German political leader on the Carter administration's reported plan to produce a neutron bomb: "a symbol of mental perversion" (Getler, 1977). And Eldridge Cleaver's former friends on Eldridge Cleaver, after learning of his shift from black radical militant to capitalist religious conservative: "schizophrenic" (Allman, 1977).

Diagnosis has also surfaced as a weapon within psychiatry. In 1964, American psychiatrists, in a poll, diagnosed as mentally ill a presidential candidate, Barry Goldwater, with whose views many of them disagreed. A decade earlier, members of the profession in supporting the Alger Hiss defense diagnosed Hiss's accuser, Whittaker Chambers, as a psychopath without ever having examined him. And the Central Intelligence Agency (CIA) understanding the power of diagnosis to discredit, made plans in 1954 to use it in covert operations (Horrock, 1977). Its hope was to administer LSD to antagonists it wished to make mad or, more to the point, wished to be diagnosed by others as mad. Under the influence of the drug, these enemies of the United States would seem psychotic and presumably be rejected or deposed by their own people.

But the most flagrant setting for the raw use of psychiatry to discredit—and, indeed, to intimidate and punish—is probably Russia. During the past decade, probably several hundred dissidents have been arrested for political trespasses, sent to psychiatrists, found mentally ill, and committed for involuntary stays at psychiatric hospitals for the criminally insane (Committee on the Judiciary, 1972; Stone, 1972; Chodoff, 1974; Amnesty International, 1975; Yeo, 1975; Grigorenko, 1976; Bloch & Reddaway, 1977; Lader, 1977; Bukovsky, 1979; Plyushch, 1979). Of these, some were truly ill (Reich, 1978a,b), but some almost surely were not (Reich, 1979a,b). To the extent that they were not, and to the extent that the diagnoses in those cases were rendered at the direct or indirect request of governmental authorities, these actions represent the worst expression of psychiatric abuse. The motivations behind the misdiagnoses were probably mixed, and in many cases the diagnoses were probably issued in full if misguided sincerity (Reich, 1978a,b). At least some may have resulted from, or been made possible by, the availability or influence of the Moscow School's overly broad and overly inclusive criteria for the diagnosis of schizophrenia. But the fact that those misdiagnoses *could* be issued, and the fact that psychiatrists were asked to examine these dissidents in the first place, also have something to do with the tempting beauty of diagnosis in all its array—not only as a means to discredit and punish but also to dehumanize, to transform social deviance into medical illness, to reassure, and to explain.

Comment. Succumbing to the nonmedical beauty of diagnosis puts one at risk, whether layman or psychiatrist, for being injured by that beauty. For years people have been coming to psychiatrists to circumvent the law, seeking diagnoses to help them get abortions or evade the military draft. Psychiatrists often saw little danger in such humanitarian deeds and willingly responded to the requests. But the danger was there, and one need only look to Russia to appreciate its extreme potential.

Things went awry in that country because a powerful tool was just too attractive and subject to misuse to be protected from such misuse; the fear of governmental power was too great, the respect for law too weak, the diagnostic scheme too broad, and the opportunities for self-deception by ordinary bureaucrats and well-trained psychiatrists too available. But the same attraction to diagnosis, the same appreciation of its multiple beauties, exists in the West, too. Though our laws have so far protected us from succumbing to Russia's fate, the law itself has a certain weakness for diagnosis, tends to be partial to its charms, and is exquisitely susceptible to its inroads. Eventually, psychiatrists will have to understand that diagnosis plays a powerful, varied, and unrecognized role in the lives of all persons, not excluding psychiatrists, and that all abuses of diagnoses—ultimately, all abuses of psychiatry—are a psychiatric problem in considerable measure because they are a human problem and probably stem less from professional corruption than from the needs and vulnerabilities of us all.

Naturally, psychiatrists must be expected not to misdiagnose knowingly. But in order to avert nonpurposeful misdiagnoses, they must come to appreciate the limitations of the diagnostic process itself, the capacity of diagnostic theories and schools to influence and shape psychiatric perceptions of behavior, and the inherent beauties of diagnosis that make it so enticing to use. Only the most stringent efforts by practitioners and the most serious attention by those who provide teaching and training will keep psychiatrists from yielding unknowingly to those beauties—indeed, will keep them from failing to recognize that the temptations even exist.

References

Allman, T. D. (1977), The 'rebirth' of Eldridge Cleaver. *New York Times Magazine*, January 16, p. 10.

Amnesty International (1975), *Prisoners of Conscience in the USSR: Their Treatment and Conditions*. London: Amnesty International Publications.

Anderson, J. & Whitten, L. (1976), Saudis suspect an Iran-U.S. plot. *Washington Post*, September 17, p. D-19.

Astrachan, B. M., Harrow, M., Adler, D., et al. (1972), A checklist for the diagnosis of schizophrenia. *Brit. J. Psychiatry* 121:529–539.

Astrup, C. & Odegard, O. (1970), Continued experiments in psychiatric diagnosis. *Acta Psychiatr. Scand.* 456:180–212.

Babigian, H. M., Gardner, E. A., Miles, H. C., et al. (1965), Diagnostic consistency and change in a follow-up study of 1,215 patients. *Am. J. Psychiatry* 121:895–901.

Balint, M. (1957), *The Doctor, His Patient, and the Illness.* New York: International Universities Press.

Berry, J. D. & Egan, J. (1977), Alleged embezzling, maneuvering in moviedom. *Washington Post,* December 25, p. A-1.

Bloch, S. & Reddaway, P. (1977), *Psychiatric Terror.* New York: Basic Books.

Brody, J. E. (1974a), Inquiry at cancer center finds fraud in research. *New York Times,* May 25.

———— (1974b), Scientist denies cancer research fraud. *New York Times,* May 29.

Bukovsky, V. (1979), *To Build a Castle: My Life as a Dissenter,* translated by Michael Scammell. New York: Viking Press.

Cantwell, D. P., Russell, A. T., Mattison, R., et al. (1979), A comparison of DSM-II and DSM-III in the diagnosis of childhood psychiatric disorders. I. Agreement with expected diagnosis. *Arch. Gen. Psychiatry* 36:1208–1213.

Chodoff, P. (1974), Involuntary hospitalization of political dissenters in the Soviet Union. *Psychiatric Opinion* 11:5–19.

Colen, D. (1975), Drug for sex offenders called success. *Washington Post,* December 5.

Committee on the Judiciary (1972), *Abuse of Psychiatry for Political Repression in the Soviet Union.* Hearing before the Subcommittee to Investigate the Administration of the Internal Security Act and Other Internal Security Laws of the Committee on the Judiciary, United States Senate, Ninety-Second Congress, Second Session. Washington, D.C.: U.S. Government Printing Office.

Evans, R. & Novak, R. (1979), Brother Billy: Political blunders. *Washington Post,* March 2.

Farrell, W. (1978), The furor surrounding Begin: He fights harder and doesn't budge. *New York Times,* July 25.

Fish, F. (1962), *Schizophrenia.* Bristol, England: John Wright and Sons.

Fowler, R. C., Tsuang, M. T., Cadoret, R. J., et al. (1975), Non-psychotic disorders in the families of process schizophrenics. *Acta Psychiatr. Scand.* 51:153–160.

Getler, M. (1977), Bonn party aide calls U.S. bomb a "perversion." *Washington Post,* July 18, p. A-1.

Grigorenko, P. (1976), *The Grigorenko Papers: Writings by General P. G. Grigorenko and Documents on His Case.* London: C. Hurst; Boulder, Colorado: Westview Press.

Gup, T. (1979), Brooding replaces clowning. *Washington Post*, February 25, p. A-1.

Hite, C. (1974), Bridging the U.S.-Soviet psychiatric gap. *Psychiatric News*, 9 (pt. 1): 6–17, 19 (pt. 2):30–32, 40.

Holland, J. (1975), Draft of pilot study of joint classification of schizophrenia. Psychiatric Research Institute USSR/Academy of Medical Sciences and NIMH/USA. Unpublished.

———— (1977a), Schizophrenia in the Soviet Union. In: *Annual Review of Research in Schizophrenia*, ed. R. Cancro. New York.

———— (1977b), 'State' hospitals in the USSR: A model of governmental psychiatric care. In: *Future Roles of State Hospitals*, ed. J. Zusman & B. Bertsen. pp. 373–385. Toronto: Lexington Books (D.C. Health).

Holland, J. & Shakhmatova-Pavlova, I. V. (1974), Concept and classification of schizophrenia in the Soviet Union. Unpublished.

Horrock, N. M. (1977), Drug tested by C. I. A. on mental patients. *New York Times*, August 3, p. A-1.

Jaspers, K. (1910), Eifersuchtswahn: Ein Beitrag zur Frage "Entwicklung einer Personlichkeit oder Prozess." *Z. Gesamte Neurol. Psychiatrie* 1:567.

Katz, M. M., Cole, J. O., & Lower, H. A. (1969), Studies of the diagnostic process: The influence of symptom perception, past experience, and ethnic background on diagnostic decisions. *Am. J. Psychiatry* 125:937–947.

Kety, S. S., Rosenthal, D., Wender, P. H., et al. (1968), The types and prevalence of mental illness in the biological adoptive families of adopted schizophrenics. In: *The Transmission of Schizophrenia*, ed. D. Rosenthal & S. S. Kety, pp. 345–362. London: Pergamon Press.

———— (1975), Mental illness in the biological and adoptive families of adopted individuals who have become schizophrenic: A preliminary report based upon psychiatric interviews. In: *Genetic Research in Psychiatry*, ed. R. Fieve, D. Rosenthal, & H. Brill, pp. 147–165. Baltimore: Johns Hopkins University Press.

———— (1978a), The biologic and adoptive families of adopted individuals who became schizophrenic: Prevalence of mental illness and other characteristics. In: *The Nature of Schizophrenia*, ed. L. C. Wynne, R. L. Cromwell, & S. Matthysse, pp. 25–37. New York: John Wiley.

Kety, S. S., Wender, P. H., & Rosenthal, D. (1978b), Genetic relationships within the schizophrenia spectrum: Evidence from adoption studies. In: *Critical Issues in Psychiatric Diagnosis*, ed. R. L. Spitzer & D. F. Klein., pp. 213–223. New York: Raven Press.

Khomeini, R. (1979), The world is not on your side. *Washington Post*, November 22, p. A-23.

Khrushchev, N. (1970), *Khrushchev Remembers*, tr. and ed. Strobe Talbott. Boston: Little, Brown.

Lader, M. (1977), *Psychiatry on Trial.* Harmondsworth, England: Penguin Books.

Langfeldt, G. (1960), Diagnosis and prognosis of schizophrenia. *Proc. Roy. Soc. Med.* 53:1047–1052.

Lenin, V. I. (1951–1967), *Sochineniya* (Works), 4th ed. Moscow State Political Literature Publishing House.

———— (1975), Letter to Gorky of July 31, 1919. Quoted in: Navrozov, L., *The Education of Lev Navrozov*, p. 164. New York: Harper's Magazine Press.

Levene, H. I. (1971), Acute schizophrenia: Clinical effects of the labelling process. *Arch. Gen. Psychiatry* 25:215–222.

Lifton, R. J. (1973), *Home from the War.* New York: Simon and Schuster.

Mandelstam, N. (1970), *Hope against Hope.* New York: Atheneum.

Mehlman, P. (1952), The reliability of psychiatric diagnoses. *J. Abnormal Soc. Psychology* 47:577–578.

Mitgang, H. (1979), Greene calls profile of him in New Yorker inaccurate. *New York Times*, May 12.

Muller-Hegemann, D. (1968), Psychotherapy in the German Democratic Republic. In: *Psychiatry in the Communist World*, ed. A. Kiev, pp. 51–70. New York: Science House.

Myer, J. K. & Reter, D. J. (1979), Sex reassignment: Follow-up. *Arch. Gen. Psychiatry* 36:1010–1015.

Nadzharov, R. A. (1972), Course forms. In: *Schizophrenia*, ed. A. V. Snezhnevsky, pp. 16–76. Moscow: Meditsina.

Newsweek (1979), The stewardess and the "witch." April 30, p. 31.

New York Times (July 16, 1976), Libya helping terrorists with arms and training.

———— (November 10, 1979), p. 8.

Overall, J. E. & Hollister, L. E. (1979), Comparative evaluation of research diagnostic criteria for schizophrenia. *Arch. Gen. Psychiatry* 36:1198–1205.

Pasamanick, B., Dinitz, S., & Lefton, L. (1959), Psychiatric orientation in relation to diagnosis and treatment. *Am. J. Psychiatry* 116:127–132.

Plutchik, R., Conte, H. & Landau, H. (1972), A comparison of symptom evaluations by psychiatrists and social workers. *Hosp. Community Psychiatry* 23:13–14.

Plyushch, L. (1979), *History's Carnival*, with a contribution by Tatyana Plyushch, ed. and tr. Marco Carynnyk. New York: Harcourt Brace Jovanovich.

Quinn, S. (1979), Rosalynn's journey. *Washington Post*, July 25, p. B-1.

Randal, J. C. (1979), Role in U.N. session builds confidence among Palestinians. *Washington Post*, January 12.

Reich, W. (1975), The spectrum concept of schizophrenia: Problems for diagnostic practice. *Arch. Gen. Psychiatry* 32:489–498.

———— (1976a), Brainwashing, psychiatry and the law. *New York Times*, May 29, p. 23.

———— (1976b), Brainwashing, psychiatry and the law. *Psychiatry* 39:400–403.

———— (1976c), The schizophrenia spectrum: A genetic concept. *J. Nerv. Ment. Dis.* 162:3–12.

———— (1978a), Soviet psychiatry on trial. *Commentary*, January, pp. 40–48.

———— (1978b), Diagnosing Soviet dissidents. *Harper's Magazine*, August, pp. 31–37.

———— (1979a), Grigorenko gets a second opinion. *New York Times Magazine*, May 13, 18ff.

———— (1979b), Kazanetz, schizophrenia and Soviet psychiatry. *Arch. Gen. Psychiatry* 36:1029–1030.

———— (1980), The diagnosis of everyday life. *Harper's Magazine*, July, pp. 6–8.

Rieder, R. O. (1978), The schizophrenia spectrum. Presented at the 131st Annual Meeting of the American Psychiatric Association, May 8–12.

Rollins, N. (1972), *Child Psychiatry in the Soviet Union.* Cambridge, Mass.: Harvard University Press.

Rosenthal, D. (1963), *The Genain Quadruplets.* New York: Basic Books.

Rosenthal, D., Wender, P. H., Kety, S. S., et al. (1968), Schizophrenic's offspring reared in adoptive homes. In: *The Transmission of Schizophrenia*, ed. S. S. Kety, D. Rosenthal, & P. H. Wender, pp. 377–391. Oxford: Pergamon Press.

———— (1971), The adopted away offspring of schizophrenics. *Am. J. Psychiatry* 128:302–306.

Rumke, H. C. (1950), Signification de la phénoménologie dans l'étude clinique des délirants. *Psychopathologie Générale* 1:125.

Scheff, T. (1966), *Being Mentally Ill: A Sociological Theory.* Chicago: Aldine.

Schram, M. (1979), The troubled times of a different Billy Carter. *Washington Post*, February 25, p. A-1.

Sinclair, W. (1979), After the upheaval: Who's running what? *Washington Post*, July 21, p. A-1.

Snezhnevsky, A. V. (1971a), Symptom, syndrome, disease: A clinical method in psychiatry. In: *The World Biennial of Psychiatry and Psychotherapy*, ed. S. Arieti, vol. 1, pp. 151–164.

———— (1971b), The symptomatology, clinical forms and nosology of schizophrenia. In: *Modern Perspectives in World Psychiatry*, ed. J. G. Howells, pp. 423–447. New York: Brunner/Mazel.

Snezhnevsky, A. V. & Vartanyan, M. (1970), The forms of schizophrenia and their biological correlates. In: *Biochemistry, Schizophrenia, and Affective Illness,* ed. H.E. Himwich, pp. 1–28. Baltimore: Williams and Wilkins.

Stone, I. F. (1972), Betrayal by psychiatry. *New York Review of Books,* February 10, pp. 7–14.

Temerlin, M. K. (1970), Diagnostic bias in community mental health. *Community Mental Health J.* 6:110–117.

Washington Post (November 24, 1977), p. A-39, Mrs. Sakharov flies home.

⸺ (July 22, 1979), p. A-6, Weicker suggests Carter not run.

Wender, P. H., Rosenthal, D., Kety, S. S., et al. (1974), Crossfostering: Research strategy for clarifying the role of genetic and experimental factors in the etiology of schizophrenia. *Arch. Gen. Psychiatry* 30: 121–128.

World Health Organization (1973), *Report of the International Pilot Study of Schizophrenia,* vol. 1. Geneva: WHO.

Yeo, C. (Summer, 1975), The abuse of psychiatry in the U.S.S.R.: The evidence. *Index on Censorship,* vol. 4, no. 2.

Zigler, E. & Phillips, L. (1961), Psychiatric diagnosis and symptomatology. *J. Abnormal Soc. Psychology* 63:69–75.

Chapter 3

Ethical Issues in Psychiatric Research on Communities: A Case Study of the Community Mental Health Center Program

ROBERT MICHELS

SPENCER ETH

Epidemiology is the study of the physical, biological, and social environment in relation to the development, distribution, and severity of disease. Its origins stem from the interest of physicians in the devastating outbreaks of illness that periodically ravaged populations. Today we recognize these as "epidemics" and give credit to John Snow for his successful inquiry into the cause of an epidemic of acute gastroenteritis in 19th-century London. Scientific epidemiology has developed with continued regard for the patterns of disease parameters (incidence, prevalence, etc.) and growing concern for active prevention and treatment—in the tradition of Snow's dismantling of the Broad Street water pump, a therapeutic intervention that preceded the germ theory of disease.

Psychiatric epidemiology is the division of epidemiology that deals primarily with issues of mental health and illness. As with general epidemiology, it had its roots in the study of various epidemics of mental disorders and has since expanded into a wider discipline involved with large-scale surveys of psychiatric symptoms and diseases, with investigations into the nature of etiology and risk factors, and with studies of mental health services and related social policy decisions. Extensive recent interest in the last area has been generated by the community mental health movement and its corollary, so-called deinstitutionalization. Throughout, the essence of epidemiology remains centered on activities directed toward groups of people or communities, rather than individual persons or patients.

The border between routine and/or best available care on the one hand and clinical research on the other is often indistinct in part because these two activities may be carried out by the same practitioner and may coexist in the treatment of an individual patient. For example, a depressed patient receiving standard pharmacological treatment may also be monitored for antidepressant blood level for correlation with clinical response. Whenever a procedure is designated a "trial" for possible wider application, or is part of an experimental design incorporating data collection and analysis, then most would agree that formal research, with all its attendant implications, is involved. "The essence of an experiment is that we deliberately apply certain procedures for the purpose of measuring their effects" (Cochran, 1955). Uncertainty arises in the borderline category of clinical activities designated as "innovative." In these cases, advanced or novel techniques that deviate, however slightly, from common practice are employed in the course of therapy. When more than minimal risk or more than a small number of patients is involved, a research protocol is usually developed. However, it has not been customary to regard innovative changes in health delivery systems in the same way. The trial of a new drug in a small group of patients is much more likely to be regarded as psychiatric research than is the closing of a state-wide network of mental hospitals and the discharge of chronic patients into the community.

The World Medical Association has recognized the need for a broad concept of research in its definition of an experiment: ". . . an act whereby the investigator deliberately changes the internal or external environment in order to observe the effects of the change" (McNeil et al., 1970). One could argue that an innovative health delivery system is one such deliberate change and warrants the same scientific scrutiny as a new drug or any other putative advance in medical treatment awaiting proof of safety and efficacy. The community mental health center program was selected for a specific case study of psychiatric research on communities. We will examine some of the ethical issues raised by the shift in mental health policy inherent in the community mental health movement and the deinstitutionalization of psychiatric patients, focusing our attention on the unique ethical problems that emerge in community level interventions.

The United States community mental health movement had its genesis early in this century. In 1913, Adolph Meyer advocated a comprehensive, multidisciplinary system of psychiatric prevention, treatment, and aftercare centered in the community (Weston, 1975). Little was done concretely until the 1920s when the Commonwealth Fund supported the development of a series of child guidance centers (Alexander & Selesnick 1966). Following World War II, mental hygiene outpatient clinics were established in many cities, although the majority of services for the mentally ill remained in mental hospitals. Conditions in these facilities were frequently deplorable. The journalist Albert Deutsch documented patient neglect in the 1940s (Deutsch, 1946). By the late 1950s the criticism of state hospital psychiatric treatment was beginning to lead to reform, with growing interest in the significance of the hospital milieu, attempts to integrate hospital treatment with family and community programs, and, of course, the development of more effective pharmacotherapy.

An important landmark of this era was the report of the Commission on Mental Health and Mental Illness (1961) whose findings and recommendations were supported by President John Kennedy in his Address to the Nation delivered February 2, 1963. He proposed a radical goal that ". . . most of [the] mentally ill are to be successfully and quickly treated in their own communities and returned to a useful place in society . . . [and to] reduce the number of patients now under custodial care by 50 percent or more" (Kennedy, 1963). Congress incorporated these goals into the Community Mental Health Center Act of 1963 (Public Law 88–164) which funded construction of community mental health centers based on an inventory of facilities and a survey of need. Need was to be determined by the extent of mental illness and emotional disorder, with consideration of poverty, substance abuse, and special interest constituencies. Staffing and further construction grants were allocated through subsequent congressional amendments (Public Law 89–105, 1965; Public Law 91–211, 1970; Public Law 94–63, 1975; etc.).

A dramatic reversal of public policy was supposed to occur. Instead of the mentally ill being confined to distant state hospitals, they were to be cared for while residing in their own homes, if possible, and certainly within their own communities. The Governor of New York expressed the new ideology: "A mental patient's well-being and his chance for recovery are best served if he can be treated at home while maintaining his ties with family and community" (Rockefeller, 1965). In addition, the domain of the community mental health center was to extend far beyond the realm of the traditional psychiatric patient. These centers were also mandated to promote the positive mental health of all community members through preventive, consultative, and educational programs. By July 1975 there were 507 community mental health centers serving over 80 million Americans. According to the former director of the National Institute of Mental Health, the community mental health center program ". . . has had a significant impact on the directions of health and mental health service delivery" (Brown & Goldstein, 1978).

In effect, there has been a major transformation in the system of mental health care delivery to about a third of the nation's citizens. This process has been designed, sanctioned, and supported by the federal government. Without formal recognition, the community mental health center movement has become our most ambitious psychiatric epidemiological research project—a massive attempt ". . . to systematically introduce planned innovations in service delivery and to assess their effects in reaching target populations that were identified as underserved by the results of field epidemiological and social area studies" (Struening, 1977).

The research aspect of the community mental health center program is intrinsic to the nature of its goals and exists regardless of the presence or absence of a formal experimental design. At its inception this program was intended as an innovative approach to meeting the mental health needs of the United States. Ongoing evaluation was deemed critical to assess its performance and the desirability of continued funding, although no truly controlled studies were instituted. In retrospect, provisions for more rigorous scientific monitoring of outcome would certainly have yielded valuable data, but their absence does not negate the research nature of this large-scale trial of an innovative psychiatric service delivery model. The absence of controls and other methodological refinements may lead to inferior research, but it is research nonetheless.

Ethics of Community Research

There are several categories of ethical problems that arise in the context of community research. Familiar ones include issues of subject privacy, confidentiality, information storage, etc. As important as these topics are, they are not unique to a discussion of community mental health centers and are adequately reviewed elsewhere. One question that emerges in new terms in the consideration of community mental health centers concerns the sponsorship of community research: What are the ethical issues involved in the approval and public support of a large-scale innovative community program? The complexity of this question becomes clearer when one examines the customary manner in which research ideas are transformed into clinical human subject experiments.

A typical small-scale research project begins with an investigator's interest and proceeds with the preparation of a protocol, the review and approval of the protocol by an institutional review board, the quest for funding, and finally the conduct of the research. The funding decision is usually made by a review panel of experts who assess the competitive worth of each protocol vying for scarce financial resources. If the proposal has survived the journey through the initiating department, institutional review board, and funding agency review, the project can then be implemented. This elaborate procedure interposes a series of sieves through which proposals must pass before a project begins. As always, the clinical investigator defines what the project intends to do but no longer determines whether it will be done. That decision is now shared with other authorities.

This mechanism of assigning the responsibility for the protection of subjects from experimental risk to the institutional review board and the responsibility for distributing scarce resources to the funding agency ensures maximal ethical scrutiny. Both panels must consider the protocol's scientific merit, for the scientific value of the research is an important factor in determining the acceptable level of risk. Both also consider ethical questions, but their ethical domains differ substantially. The institutional review board is primarily concerned with patient/subject protection from experimental risk. No research can be approved if it exposes the participants to danger without appropriate personal and community advantage. The institutional review board's decision requires a close analysis of the impact of the research on the participants. The funding agency's ethical agenda focuses on the potential value of the scientific findings. Its task is to distribute scarce resources so as to increase the likelihood of significant benefit to society. The agency's priority is to represent the needs and wishes of the population at large. This sequential system of review, monitoring both the "means" and the "ends" of every protocol, is standard for small-scale investigations.

The large-scale community mental health center program did not follow this combined institutional review board and funding agency review route. No explicit consideration was given to the protection of the patients/subjects or to whether the proposed plan was best suited to achieve the desired goals. The Community Mental Health Center Act of 1963 was adopted by Congress, not by a panel of experts, with a budget allocated from general revenues. This exceptional situation arose because large-scale changes in our mental health care delivery system required a huge financial outlay, the funds for which were not available within the traditional research agencies.

This shift from the scientific to the political arena underscores the dual nature of all research, simultaneously both scientific inquiry and political action. When research is in a controversial area, like community mental health, its political significance in the broader sense may dwarf its importance as inquiry. The method required for securing approval and funding for large-scale political programs may conflict with the customary procedures for insuring review of the ethical aspects of medical research.

It is undesirable for researchers to avoid inquiry into controversial areas, inappropriate for society to relinquish its influence on and regulation of research with large-scale political significance, and probably unethical to ignore the fact that research in controversial areas is inquiry and to treat it solely as political action.

We are left with the need for appropriate ways for society to participate in decisions concerning the political, ethical, and scientific aspects of community research.

The Community and Scientific Review

A crucial issue is how the community can best participate in the scientific review process. The model that has evolved in the regulation of small-scale investigations seems appealing. Elected representatives responsible for allocation of public resources distribute money to various specific funding agencies that reflect the concerns of the community. Final decisions on specific projects involve experts who have the requisite knowledge to evaluate the relative scientific merit and value of competing proposals. It is their charge to select those that have the greatest probability of fulfilling the community's goals.

By extrapolation, large-scale projects could be handled in the same fashion. The general community could be involved in monitoring the boundaries of scientific decision-making without direct control over its content. This would recognize that the community and its general (political) representatives are not sufficiently competent to make decisions about the scientific aspects of research projects and should defer such decisions to selected elite groups. This is not an unusual notion; there are many decisions the community-at-large is ill-suited to make. For example, they are not prepared to determine what dose of chlorpromazine to administer to a person having a psychotic episode. They are no better able to decide whether a particular project has sufficient scientific merit to warrant support. The fact that the large-scale proposal involves many millions of people and huge sums of money does not increase the community's competence; it only underscores the importance of choosing goals carefully and rigorously evaluating options. The scale of the project may determine its political importance but does not ensure that the political process will lead to a scientifically appropriate or ethically acceptable decision.

In the case of providing psychiatric services for the nation, the Congress, as the duly elected representatives of the people, would choose to place emphasis on community mental health and to provide funds for developing and delivering psychiatric care in the community. A separate, autonomous group of experts would be assigned the task of choosing the specific, most desirable community mental health proposal from among all those submitted. This intervening group would be elitist in the sense of having the expertise necessary to evaluate competing proposals. In this structure the community's general representatives make the value judgments—more funds for community mental health in place of traditional hospital-based psychiatric services—while a panel of authorities decides which of the competing projects is most likely to succeed in satisfying the community's wishes and, therefore, should be awarded the funds. The absence of that intervening structure renders the technical decision-making process vulnerable to the ills of political whim and adversarial pressures.

Ethical Problems of Community Psychiatry

A second ethical issue, fundamental to the community mental health center program, is analogous to the concerns of the institutional review board in small-scale research. It relates to the moral legitimacy of the decision to transfer the locus of psychiatric treatment from the state hospital to the patient's own home and community. While most parties believed that there would be benefits for the identified patient, the probable impact on family and neighbors was more controversial. The actual effects have been complex and not always as predicted.

The major rationale for the community mental health movement was well described by its advocate, Gruenberg (1969): "Most descriptions of the nature of psychoses continue to identify chronic disorganized behavior, combativeness, suicidal tendencies, deterioration, and vegetable existence as direct manifestations of certain psychotic disorders. Yet when patients with these psychotic disorders are treated in comprehensive, community-based psychiatric services which provide continuity of care, these behavioral distortions develop much more rarely, and when they do these patterns almost always last only a short time." This statement claims substantial clinical benefit for patients treated in community mental health centers where there is opportunity for both secondary and tertiary prevention and the patient is spared the additional psychosocial burden of stigma.

The community mental health movement has been applauded as a "humanitarian vision that has moved concerned professionals and laypersons to work toward the reintegration of the mentally disabled into a society that historically has preferred to relegate them to the dehumanizing environment of a warehouse" (Lander, 1975). This reflects the proposition that deinstitutionalization and community care afford the psychiatric patient a greater degree of freedom, which has inherent value beyond its clinical advantage. At question, however, is whether the psychiatric patient in the community is actually more free. Much depends on the patient's psychological capacities: awareness of life's options and ability to deliberate and choose among them. Freedom has little meaning if the patient's environment has a paucity of alternatives from which to choose. The patient also needs the will to act and the opportunity to act without coercion. It is far from clear that the majority of chronic psychiatric patients in the community are truly "free." Yet the circumstances of even the best mental hospital also deprive patients of many aspects of personal freedom.

A further nonclinical benefit claimed by community mental health proponents was a projected financial saving. They argued that deinstitutionalization would result in huge budget cuts. Tragically, it soon became clear that this could only be assured by the simultaneous nondevelopment of substantial community care resources, although the public rhetoric had emphasized community care. From a pragmatic political viewpoint, the cost-savings claims were very persuasive. "We believe that a comprehensive local mental health program that functions effectively is in fact an inexpensive health delivery system when compared to the traditional methods of using distant state hospitals for acute psychiatric care" (Stubblebine & Decker, 1971). This appeal to legislative parsimony was dangerously seductive. It helped to sell community mental health centers to a cost-conscious Congress and further implied that expenses could be continuously trimmed without diminishing quality. Funding problems are today the decisive issue that threatens the survival of the community mental health center program.

Some of the more enthusiastic advocates of community mental health maintained that the presence of a community mental health center and wider community access to psychiatric care would exert a positive and preventive effect on the mental health of the community. There has been much debate on which, if any, interventions have a primary preventive impact on the population at large (Roberts, 1968). Even more controversial have been attempts to promote "positive" mental health.

Psychiatrists are acknowledged to have expertise in the diagnosis and treatment of mental illness, but any claim to a corresponding knowledge of positive mental health is questionable. It is this claim that has led to community psychiatry's involvement in civil rights, sex education, ghetto community organization, and the Head Start program. One could argue about whether each of these activities helps to assure the psychosocial prerequisites of enhanced mental health (Gottesfeld, 1972).

From the start, recognized harms, as well as benefits, were associated with community treatment of psychiatric patients, particularly if "community" is equated with "home" (Hoenig & Hamilton, 1966; Tucker, 1966). Some patients, for whom life in the community had been pathogenic, would not benefit from living at home. "It is almost the rule that it is not merely helpful but actually essential (in the launching of treatment) to lift the patient out of all his familiar settings. This is not new wisdom; it is so old that it seems to have been forgotten" (Grad & Sainsbury, 1968). Another group of patients was at risk from a precipitous policy of deinstitutionalization. These were those chronic state hospital patients who could be discharged only with pain and difficulty from the hospitals that had become their homes.

A serious objection to the community mental health movement was based on the deleterious effects of community treatment on the patient's family. Although some families are capable of caring for an ill relative, others are less able to cope with the burden of psychiatric illness in a spouse or parent (Kubie, 1968; Williams et al., 1973; Creer & Wing, 1974). Ironically, this can lead to a community mental health prescription of hospitalization rather than community care, as suggested by Rutter (1966) when he commented: "If the cost of keeping a parent in the community is the development of psychiatric disorder in the children, then it may be too high."

Despite the interpersonal pathogenic potential of community psychiatric treatment, many families prefer having the patient at home. In one large study of schizophrenics maintained in the community (Brown et al., 1966), the patients' relatives complained of poor health, financial difficulties, and social restrictions; nevertheless 75 percent of the families actively welcomed the patient in the home and another 15 percent became increasingly accepting. Fewer than 10 percent rejected the patient or actively sought psychiatric hospitalization. These positive feelings expressed for maintaining patients in their families reveal a considerable reservoir of tolerance and concern, which is therapeutically beneficial for the patient. The inherent caring abilities of such families can be enhanced greatly by comprehensive community services. Programs that provide home visits and social services are particularly helpful to both patient and family (Langsley et al., 1971). The addition of a day hospital component can offer a significant relief to the family, thereby lifting much of the burden of community treatment without sacrificing the advantages of community care (Byrne, 1974). A good treatment plan for the patient can be a good treatment plan for relatives as well, if sufficient extramural aid is available. The community mental health center was designed to supply this full range of services to all community members, patient and family alike; this has always been its mandate. "A society which has, for its own reasons, decided that the long-stay hospital is not the place in which schizophrenics should be treated owes all possible skilled advice and support to those who have taken over the responsibility" (*Lancet*, 1974).

Unfortunately the provisions for aftercare support of indigent psychiatric patients are often grossly inadequate. The public has expressed its concern for the social effects of the psychiatric nomads visibly congregating in the streets. Its outrage has been expressed loudly by the residents of the Upper West Side of Manhattan, whose neighborhood has become the site of single-room-occupancy (SRO) hotels catering to deinstitutionalized patients. The lack of appropriate supervision and ongoing treatment accentuates the problems these disabled citizens face in finding productive activities and in attempting to assimilate into the community. Without sufficient financial support these problems multiply to the detriment of patients, neighborhoods, and community mental health centers alike.

In summary, it would seem that there are usually both clinical and nonclinical benefits for the patient in community care, while the impact on the patient's family is more often deleterious. Also, particularly for patients without families, the negative impact on the neighborhood is often striking (Arnhoff, 1975). Any course of action that produces conflicting effects raises concerns about the manner in which the advantages and disadvantages are distributed. What are the differences between the community mental health center program and the state mental hospital system in the apportionment of benefits and harm?

Behind any discussion of the choice of a specific mental health policy looms an unarticulated question of competing models of ethical theory. For example, some would argue that institutionalization of the mentally ill is preferable because it protects the family and neighborhood from the burdens and risks of community care. The proponents of this policy might not realize that the foundation of their belief is the contemporary ethical theory of rule utilitarianism (Frankena, 1973). The utilitarian approach to social justice tends to favor the greater good for the larger number. With society as a reference point, utilitarians would argue that the largest number of people are served by the distant incarceration of the mentally ill. Since no one can accurately predict whether a given citizen will become a psychiatric patient or remain well, there is no *a priori* discrimination in a hospital-based system. Further, since there are far more healthy community residents who benefit from the hospitalization of the few who are ill, the moral calculus points towards hospitalization.

The position favoring a community mental health center policy might be supported by a different ethical theory—one that emphasizes concern for the distribution of sacrifices imposed by a mental hospital-based system. It would argue that the major burdens of an institutional system of care fall on the patients who are already the unfortunate victims of mental illness. Justice would be better served by a policy that allows patients already afflicted by mental illness to be compensatorily rewarded by a system that favors their care. In this way the interests of the well majority are overridden in order to provide advantages for the ill minority. The philosopher Rawls (1971) convincingly advocated a procedure for producing this outcome.

In Rawls' procedure, a community member is asked to imagine the following hypothetical situation. He is to act reasonably but is to decide on a plan while cloaked in a "veil of ignorance." That means that he is completely unaware of his own age, social status, natural assets and liabilities, interests, etc. He does, of course, have a general knowledge of human nature, including the values of personal well-being, functional capacity, and the happiness of fulfilling life's goals. For example, the goal of this thought experiment would be for the community member to choose a plan for psychiatric care for the mentally ill—either community or hospital-based. He is assumed to have a natural and typical self-interest but will choose fairly and without exploitation since he must make the decision without knowing whether he himself is, in fact, mentally ill or not.

Our anonymous community member, unaware of whether he is a patient, a relative, or a neighbor, must choose a plan for psychiatric care. He will certainly wish to maximize the general welfare but will be careful not to ignore the few who are most impaired since he himself might well be one of them. The greater risks of deterioration in a state hospital must weigh more heavily than the lesser risks of the smaller harms to family and neighbors in the community care of the mentally ill. Further, the certain deprivation of a patient's personal freedom within an institution is unmatched by the potential loss of liberty a relative or neighbor might suffer. Although the deleterious effects of community care are well documented, they would fall predominantly on the well relatives and more advantaged community members. Consequently anyone blind to his status as patient, family, or neighbor would seek to avoid the devastating loss of liberty and danger of deterioration involved in institutional care. However, from the family and community perspective one would demand local mental health resources to minimize the largely avoidable social sequelae of insufficient aftercare and support. In a well-funded community mental health system everyone is entitled to the same degree of personal freedom of movement. The burdens and harms of community care that do exist would tend to spare the already disadvantaged mentally ill, who would also be the recipients of the principal benefits. The intrinsic fairness of this pattern of distribution is based on the premise that the inequalities of mental illness are open to all and are of such a magnitude as to demand special consideration.

Consent

Having discussed the role of the community in assessing the scientific value of the project and in evaluating its ethical significance, we now turn to the issue of consent, which emerges when we regard the community not as monitor or reviewer but rather as subject of the research. This topic represents the application of a concept that arose in therapeutic and experimental work with individuals to the effects of the introduction of an innovative mental health delivery system for an entire population.

The concept of voluntary consent derives from case law. In 1914, Judge Benjamin Cardozo of the New York Court of Appeals held: "Every human being of adult years and sound mind has a right to determine what shall be done with his own body; and a surgeon who performs an operation without his patient's consent commits an assault, for which he is liable" (*Schloendorff v. New York Hospital*, 1914). This constituted a successful challenge to the assumption of an unspoken consent by the patient, consistent with the common belief that it is the doctor's duty to do whatever he decides will benefit the patient. A consequence of the voluntary consent principle is that it broadens the domain of human subject research by establishing a process for patients to become subjects through voluntary consent. Both procedures intended to be therapeutic and those that are primarily investigative can proceed if, and only if, there is prior consent.

The further qualification that consent must be fully informed is more recent. The term "informed consent" was first used in *Natanson v. Kline,* 1960 by the Kansas Supreme Court, and since then there has been considerable disagreement as to the level of disclosure necessary to assure a valid consent. A Canadian court suggested a standard of information disclosure for use in research cases that could serve for routine medical practices as well: "The subject of medical experimentation is entitled to a full and frank disclosure of all the facts, probabilities and opinions which a reasonable man might be expected to consider before giving his consent" (*Halushka v. University of Saskatchewan*, 1965). The combined concepts of informed and voluntary consent strongly value individual autonomy as the best means of ensuring patient/subject self-determination, while allowing for a wide range of possible therapeutic/experimental activities.

Consent evolved as a means of protecting the individual from the physical dangers intrinsic in biomedical interventions of a therapeutic or experimental nature. By comparison scant attention has been paid to psychosocial risks, and there is virtually no literature concerning consent for interventions aimed at groups or communities of people.

In thinking about the problem of community consent, it is useful to examine the fringe areas of individual voluntary informed consent. The overriding importance of consent in the ideal case of the solo, competent adult is unquestioned. "We believe that informed consent is the basis of all psychiatric intervention and that without it no psychiatric intervention can be morally justified" (Redlich & Mollica, 1976). However, some situations deviate substantially from the ideal and require modifications of the usual principles. The first and most obvious example is the individual who is not and will not soon become competent to give consent.

Some mentally disabled people are not able to make rational decisions regarding their own welfare and cannot be expected personally to offer valid consent to their treatment, even if they appear to want to do so. This is a particularly difficult area, since psychiatric definitions of mental illness and legal definitions of incompetence overlap but rarely coincide. Especially problematic are those psychiatric patients involuntarily committed to the hospital who are near the border of incompetence with regard to the issue of informed consent for needed treatment (Stone, 1979). Consent is still required, but it must be given by another individual who has the duty to act in the interests of the impaired person. This consent is usually limited to therapeutic procedures and ordinarily excludes experimental or humanitarian activities (e.g., organ donation) involving risk or discomfort for which competent patients might offer voluntary informed consent. This scheme provides a mechanism for restricted third party consent, often through a court appointed guardian.

A comparable scheme exists for another class of persons deemed incompetent to render consent: children, younger than some designated age, who are considered unable to act rationally in their own best interest. Here, too, third party consent, usually parental, is allowed to substitute for individually given consent for treatment. This has been termed vicarious, or proxy, consent (McCormick et al., 1974) and is deemed consistent with the child's personal welfare.

Also, for some people, temporarily unable to give consent, therapeutic activities are allowed to proceed at once. For example, in emergency conditions with unconscious victims, physicians are permitted to perform needed procedures without delay. Consent may be impossible if the patient is not responsive and next of kin are not accessible. The notion of presumed consent, in which it is assumed that the injured party would consent to a life-saving intervention if able, authorizes the physician's actions.

A less dramatic example is the patient who has given specific voluntary informed consent for an operative procedure. While the patient is unconscious, the surgeon discovers some other condition that could easily be ameliorated. The courts have held that to expose the patient to the additional inconvenience and risk of a second operation for the sole purpose of obtaining prior consent is unnecessary if the vast majority of similar patients would be expected to consent. This risks violating the wishes of that small minority of patients who idiosyncratically would refuse to consent to the additional procedure, however useful or safe.

A corollary situation is the implicit consent that governs the conduct of physical examinations. Physicians may not outline in advance all the components of their usual examination. Rather they may proceed in a gentle, careful, and often educational manner, with the unspoken understanding that patient cooperation is tantamount to consent. These cases of presumed, implied, and implicit consent refer to activities for the patient's direct benefit. It is nowhere suggested that bypassing voluntary informed consent can be employed in nontherapeutic experimentation (Fried, 1974).

All these alternatives to voluntary consent for competent adults are intended for rare or exceptional circumstances. The overwhelming majority of cases require the standard rule of disclosure of all material facts pertinent to the condition and its recommended treatment. All common risks, and even remote risks if sufficiently serious, must be described. However, there has been a growing backlash to this demand for complete openness and honesty in the doctor-patient relationship. For instance, some doctors advocate a policy of not divulging the diagnosis and prognosis to certain cancer patients if it is believed the patient would be unable to cope with the news. The courts have supported this discretionary use of therapeutic privilege.

Recently, physician-investigators have proposed widening the therapeutic privilege to encompass medical experimentation (Frost, 1979; Lofius & Fries, 1979). Their argument is two-pronged. Informed consent is a ritual devoid of meaning to the patient/subject if the content of the consent cannot be understood. In that case its value is limited to the possible protection of the investigator and the sponsoring institution from lawsuits. All too often, it is charged, the patient/subject is passively led through a consent procedure, much as a foreign tourist is shown about by a guide—neither fully understanding the other.

The second argument for dispensing with detailed consent is that it can be both a hazard to the patient/subject's health and an obstacle to the investigator's research. A patient/subject can become increasingly frightened by reading the lengthy list of risks associated with even the most common drugs and procedures. The fear may not be tempered by the reassurance that the risks are small. The patient/subject might well be suggestible enough to develop one or more of these uncomfortable or potentially dangerous side effects, even if only a placebo is given. This constitutes a negative placebo effect and imposes a significant and preventable hazard to all patients/subjects who read and take seriously the detailed risks of the investigation. Some have even suggested ironically that the investigator should obtain an informed consent before subjecting the participant to the consent form!

The trend toward more comprehensive consent procedures, besides increasing the risk of negative placebo effects, makes the task of soliciting volunteers for research more difficult. The prospective experimental subjects made uncomfortable by the consent process are less likely to participate and more likely to withdraw on the unwarranted basis of iatrogenic consent anxiety. To the extent that this is happening, research is being deterred without any substantive increment in patient/subject protection.

The refusal of competent adults to consent can sometimes be overridden by agents of society. Legal precedents dating back at least 75 years attest to the power of the state to impose actions on individuals that are designed to protect the individual patient and the public—as in the case of vaccinations (*Jacobson v. Massachusetts*, 1904)—or the public alone—as in the case of quarantine (*McGuire v. Amyx*, 1927). The requirement for consent prior to physical intervention would still hold in situations where refusal to submit does not constitute a danger but merely fails to confer a benefit. For example, no one is forced to donate a rare type of blood involuntarily. However, when the safety of society is at stake, as in communicable diseases, the state can and does compel persons to act on the state's behalf.

Community Consent

Less extreme forms of government coercion abound in the psychosocial realm where the issue is less often safety and more often public welfare. Here we are moving away from physical interventions and risks to the more extensive but less concrete activities that affect external and psychosocial environments. The cumulative effects of such activities are often spread over a large population, and may affect any single individual in a diminishing or difficult-to-detect fashion.

In the United States, elected representatives enact laws to provide for the general welfare of the citizens, while those individuals with minority views retain their basic rights through constitutional guarantees and the recourse of judicial review. Representatives at every level of government routinely sacrifice the interests of individuals for the common good of the community. For example, in order to build a new highway a cascade of infringements in necessary. The man who must relinquish his house is directly affected. Although compensated financially, he has no choice but to move, however dear his own property. His neighbors may not be displaced, but they too will experience profound and unpredictable changes in their daily lives as a result of the construction of a major thoroughfare in their vicinity. Neither the homeowner, nor his neighbors, nor other community members have the right to refuse to consent to the project. In fact, even collectively they lack the power to veto plans approved by a higher political authority. Opponents, as long as their personal physical integrity is not threatened, are overruled by the much greater mass of people whose lives are more convenienced by the new road.

Highway construction is a commonplace phenomenon whose impact has been assessed in a variety of situations. Though no one can predict exactly what changes will be wrought by a new highway in a specific neighborhood, the domain of expectable responses is small. This mirrors the issues involved in the usual practice of prescribing an approved drug with a multitude of known side effects. A particular patient may experience no untoward reaction at all, but if one does occur it would probably be one that has already been reported. Although the use of any medication new to the patient is in some sense an "experiment," it is generally considered part of the art of clinical medicine. Some large-scale public projects, unlike highway construction, fall closer to the experimental or investigative end of the intervention spectrum in the sense that they may be both new and unprecedented.

The decision to open Atlantic City, New Jersey, to casino gambling would fit that model of a novel program. All agreed that widespread effects were inevitable, but even rough estimates of the impact were disputed. Proponents and opponents of the plan debated the hoped-for benefits and feared risks, without clear evidence of either or a sense of emerging consensus. The final decision was made at a higher geopolitical level than the local community. The community residents, who are now known to have been dramatically affected, had no opportunity to give prior consent; they could only protest deleterious effects after the harm had been inflicted. The risk of psychosocial or environmental harm to a community resident may be great, while the direct impact on those who are empowered to implement such large-scale projects may be insignificant. No consent is obtained from the individuals whose lives will be directly affected by the experiment.

During the distant debate by their general representatives, each community resident has but a small voice in the decision. For example, the decision to launch the Skylab mission under NASA's auspices did not involve participation by those individuals who might have been concerned that Skylab might someday fall. The public was not privy to the details of the mission in advance, and the opportunity to supply direct feedback was nonexistent.

However, a provision mandating individual consent from everyone remotely at risk from Skylab would be clearly inappropriate. There is no available mechanism to obtain a consent from the entire citizenry of the United States or of the world. And if, hypothetically, there could be the opportunity to solicit individual consent from everyone, what if Mr. X refused to consent to Skylab being placed in orbit over his home? Could failure to obtain X's permission rule out that trajectory? One alternative is to deny X the opportunity to consent, but to provide instead the right to initiate legal action in the unlikely event that Skylab should fall and injure his person or damage his property. His concern over that possible but remote calamity would not be allowed to negate a mission of general importance. The sanctioning of a vital experiment with an infinitesimal risk of individual harm, spread over a large population, ought to be within the authority of the government, if the experiment's overall safety has been adequately established. The mechanism by which that safety should be assessed is, however, less clear.

Much recent public attention has been drawn to the controversies over nuclear-powered electrical generating plants. A crisis of public confidence in scientific technology has erupted, in part as the result of disturbing disclosures and frightening events. Nuclear energy is an exceedingly complex subject which the public associates with prospects as diverse as incendiary holocausts and limitless energy. General political representatives have relied heavily on expert testimony in developing strategies first for atomic bomb testing for national defense and then for nuclear power station construction. Secure in their specialists' advice, the politicians delegated the administration and control of nuclear energy to military professionals and to technically trained nuclear regulatory commissioners. For atomic testing in the 1950s and nuclear power in the 1970s the overall risks of human harm were initially calculated to be small and randomly distributed over large populations. However, in recent years serious questions have been raised about the validity of these estimates. The extensive open-air testing of fissionable devices in the Southwest is now being linked to significantly higher incidents of cancer in adjacent Utah populations. The Three Mile Island crisis underscored the reality that, although the odds of major accidents are small, even one such accident could produce a terrifying amount of destruction in the area surrounding the facility. Here again a relevant issue is the appropriateness of requiring individual consent from each person residing near a proposed nuclear reactor. Are the dangers of a reactor comparable to the acceptable risk of the Skylab project? Or, is the model of informed consent with the option to decline to participate more applicable in this community intervention? The answer depends in part on an accurate assessment of risk, on the availability of alternative residences, and ultimately on one's position regarding the protection of the interests of the minority.

The volatile issue of mandatory public school busing illustrates another aspect of community consent. Following the Supreme Court decision that separate, segregated education was unconstitutional, lower courts enforced integration plans requiring the busing of large numbers of children to distant public schools. Unlike with government-imposed quarantines, no argument was made that the safety of the community depended on racial integration of public schools. Rather the courts acted to ensure the right of minority students to equal educational opportunity. This placed more advantaged Caucasian children in the position of either having their own schools integrated or being transported to predominantly black schools. Once both sets of schools were fully integrated, there would no longer be a discrepancy in educational environment. Parents of white children had no option to decline to participate; their choices were limited to compliance with the integration plan, enrolling their offspring in private schools, or leaving the district. The burden of busing was imposed without consent since the benefits, assuring the constitutional rights of the minority, are agreed to be overwhelming. However, community cooperation is required for school integration to work, and although the community need not formally consent, its ongoing assent is essential.

Consent and the Community Mental Health Center Program

The large-scale community mental health center program approved by Congress allowed for the participation of some United States communities. Since the concept of community mental health was innovative and untested, there was a paucity of available information. With few facts and no readily available mechanism for community consent, one government report noted: "There is no obvious or easy way to interpret or apply the principle of informed consent in the study of large groups, subcultures, or entire societies. New ways must be devised to obtain free participation" (Executive Office of the President, 1967). Obtaining consent was especially difficult in the case of community mental health centers because they were comprised of a potpourri of services. A particular center's exact character was hard to define, as its activities blurred traditional treatment, innovative treatment, and research. Unlike the fluoridation of a community's water, the development of a community mental health center affected various groups of citizens differently. When the town's leaders decide that fluoridation is no longer experimental, but rather is a safe method of promoting dental health, the fluoride ion is added to the public water supply through legislative authority. Everyone is then exposed to the same element. The construction of community mental health centers along with the deinstitutionalization of psychiatric patients can be mandated by the public's representatives as well, but the ensuing consequences are a perplexing array of personal and social effects.

Several types of consent are relevant to community mental health centers. Consider first the issue of consent for the public at large. The majority of the community is not receiving psychiatric treatment for themselves or their families. For this community of the well, major concerns will include: (1) physical injury to nonpatients (in fact, a negligible risk); (2) the nuisance aspect of deinstitutionalization (related to the community's attitude toward psychiatrically deviant neighbors); (3) the utilization of scarce financial resources; (4) the risk of invasion of privacy, perhaps through the collection of data; (5) changes in attitudes about mental illness; and (6) the impact of the center on existing community institutions, particularly in the area of mental health. The risk to nonpatients in the community may be great but is not generally regarded as the type of risk that calls for individual informed consent. However, some alternative method is needed for confirming ongoing assent and, many would add, for providing continuing input from the general community.

The issue of consent for patients presenting to the community mental health center is, by comparison, much clearer. Like their counterparts in other clinical or research settings, these patients are expected to give individual voluntary informed consent prior to receiving treatment. They must understand what is new or risky about the treatment. An immediate question is whether the innovative nature of the treatment center itself is a pertinent fact requiring disclosure to the individual patient. A preliminary answer might suggest that such disclosure is appropriate insofar as the experience of the individual patient in the center is likely to fall outside the range of average expectable patient experiences in the community.

Once treatment has commenced, a patient expects to receive continued treatment at the general level of care in the community. A care giver has the obligation to ensure that such continued treatment is available. The patient, on the other hand, retains the option to withdraw from treatment at any time regardless of any prior commitment. In fact, this right to change or discontinue treatment is an important protection for the patient since it serves as a perpetual "market test" of the service. As long as there are other options, the patient will seek to maximize treatment benefits by choosing the best treatment available. The community mental health center should flourish only if its product is a success in the marketplace. Unfortunately, the development of community mental health centers often results in the atrophy of other, pre-existing psychiatric resources. When patients and funds shift to the new centers, other facilities may not survive the loss of income. The initial popularity of community mental health centers promoted the creation of a monopoly, thereby depriving patients of both the opportunity to register a change of mind and the protections inherent in a pluralistic system. Moreover, it denied patients the possibility of ever returning to the *status quo ante*, since their previous psychiatric facility might no longer exist.

Although the centers may have defeated their competition, they have not always been able to capture and hold their funds. In part, the centers were guilty of oversell in their claims that community psychiatric treatment could be cost-effective in reducing mental health budgets. Furthermore, the existing reimbursement mechanisms insured that adequate community care must lead to operating deficits, and there was no innovative funding scheme to complement the innovative clinical services.

Community mental health centers, an innovative experiment in medical service delivery, were forced to compete in the traditional political arena for continued funding. The centers were expected to demonstrate within a short period appropriate to political decision-making that they could deliver cost-effective services. A center, struggling to meet each annual budget, could not achieve its larger mission or prove its intrinsic worth.

Community research needs a different degree of stability and decision-making than is allotted to it in the political process. Research is a capital, not an operating, expense, the yield is long-term, and the investment is in a structure, not in an immediate product. Foundations recognize this distinction by awarding research grants for longer periods. The problem for community mental health centers was compounded by a huge front-end funding requirement for construction. The centers needed a great deal of money at the start and then stability in funding over a long period of time. Unfortunately, they managed to secure only the former, to the detriment of the overall integrity of the project design.

Most medical experiments are short-term. A new procedure

either works or it fails. This outcome then determines its future use. If an experimental medication is safe and effective, it will be marketed, and patients will continue to receive it. If not, the drug will be withdrawn, and other standard remedies will be employed. The situation with community mental health centers is different. In many settings, the centers seem to be functioning well but, although definitive data are not available, their financial support is dwindling. Yet, pre-existing psychiatric facilities have often been replaced by the centers. The patient needing treatment is confronted with a paucity of alternatives and the real possibility that the only facility available might not continue. How will the right to continue receiving treatment be honored? Tragically, this question is not moot. Reports in the literature have chronicled the demise of centers. One article (Patrick, 1979) documented the closing of an inner-city community mental health center, involving the vicious cycle of falling revenues leading to program and staff cutbacks leading to further erosion of the financial base. Uncertainty depleted everyone's coping abilities during the agonal phase of the center's existence.

Patients have a right to expect to continue treatment despite a center's financial difficulties. Premature termination of treatment threatens their health and, at times, their lives. This situation is not unlike the plight that end-stage kidney patients faced prior to the passage of the social security amendment (Public Law 92–603, 1972) guaranteeing payment for life-saving renal dialysis treatments (Rettig, 1976). One can argue that there is an analogy in the general community's right to expect that the center itself will continue once it has been developed. The argument is particularly compelling when the introduction of the center has led to the withering away of other treatment alternatives.

With the advantage of hindsight, it might be argued that our resources should have been focused on a smaller number of well-funded centers with appropriate means to evaluate what the centers really do to a community. This would have been preferable scientifically, but probably impossible politically. The program has added still another faction in the mental health arena but has not led to real advances in our knowledge about mental health delivery. Decisions involved in developing the programs were made with little regard for their ethical dimensions. A more sophisticated ethical analysis of the issues at that time might have encouraged a process that generated more knowledge, protected communities from the negative effects of the centers, and produced the slower and surer development of an effective program. Such a program might have had less initial political popularity but greater eventual positive impact on the nation's mental health and greater regard for the rights of its citizens. The question is whether the political process will tolerate and accommodate the type of ethical safeguards that have become commonplace and accepted in the more traditional scientific arena.

References

Alexander, F. G. & Selesnick, S. T. (1966), *The History of Psychiatry*, p. 377. New York: Harper & Row.

Arnhoff, F. N. (1975), Social consequences of policy toward mental illness. *Science* 188:1277–1281.

Brown, B. S. & Goldstein, H. (1978), The lightning rod of human service delivery. In: Brady, J. P. and Brodie, H. K. H.: *Controversy in Psychiatry*, ed. J. P. Brady & H. K. H. Brodie. Philadelphia: Saunders.

Brown, G. W. et al. (1966), *Schizophrenia and Social Care*. London: Oxford University Press.

Byrne, L. (1974), Home behavior of schizophrenic patients living in the community and attending a day center. *Br. J. Psychiatry* 125:20–24.

Cochran, W. G. (1955), Research techniques in the study of human beings. *Milbank Mem. Fund. Q.* 33:121–136.

Creer, C. & Wing, J. K. (1974), *Schizophrenia at Home*. London: National Schizophrenia Fellowship.

Deutsch, A. (1946), *The Mentally Ill in America: A History of Their Care and Treatment from Colonial Times*. New York: Columbia University Press.

Executive Office of the President (1967), *Privacy and Behavioral Research*. Washington, D.C.: U.S. Government Printing Office.

Frankena, W. K. (1973), *Ethics*, 2d ed., chap. 2. Englewood Cliffs, New Jersey: Prentice-Hall.

Fried, C. (1974), *Medical Experimentation: Personal Integrity and Social Policy*, chap. 2, pp. 13–43. New York: Elsevier North-Holland.

Frost, N. (1979), Consent as a barrier to research. *N. Engl. J. Med.* 300: 1271–1273.

Gottesfeld, H. (1972), *Critical Issues of Community Mental Health*. New York: Behavioral Publications.

Grad, J. & Sainsbury, P. (1968), Effects that patients have on their families in a community care and a control psychiatric service—A two year follow-up. *Br. J. Psychiatry* 114:265–278.

Gruenberg, E. M. (1969), From practice to theory. *Lancet* i:721–725.

Halushka v. University of Saskatchewan (1965), 52 W.W.R. 608, 616–617 (Sask.).

Hoenig, J. & Hamilton, M. W. (1966), The schizophrenic patient in the community and his effect on the household. *Int. J. Soc. Psychiatry* 12:165–176.

Jacobson v. Massachusetts (1904), 197 U.S. 11.

Joint Commission on Mental Illness and Health (1961), *Action for mental health*. New York: Basic Books.

Kennedy, J. F. (1963), *Message Relative to Mental Illness and Mental Retardation*, Document No. 58, 88th Congress. Washington, D.C.: U.S. Government Printing Office.

Kubie, L. S. (1968), Pitfalls of community psychiatry. *Arch. Gen. Psychiatry* 18:257–266.

Lancet (1974), ii:33, The relatives of schizophrenics (editorial).

Lander, L. (1975), Mental health con game. *Health PAC Bulletin* 65:2–25.

Langsley, D. G. et al. (1971), Avoiding mental hospital admission: A follow-up study. *Am. J. Psychiatry* 127:1391–1394.

Lofius, E. F. & Fries, J. F. (1979), Consent may be hazardous to health. *Science* 104(4388):11.

McCormick, R. A. et al. (1974), Proxy consent in the experimentation situation. *Perspect. Biol. Med.* Autumn: 2–20.

McGuire v. Amyx (1927), 317 Mo. 1061, 297 S.W. 968.

McNeil, J. N. et al. (1970), Community psychiatry and ethics. *Am. J. Orthopsychiatry* 40:22–29.

Natanson v. Kline (1960), 186 Kan. 393, 350 P. 2d 1093. Clarified and rehearing denied, 187 Kan. 186, 354 P. 2d 670 (1960).

Patrick, J. (1979), Staff reaction to the closing of a community mental health center. *Hosp. Community Psychiatry* 30:259–262.

Rawls, J. (1971), *A Theory of Justice*. Cambridge, Mass.: Harvard University Press.

Redlich, F. & Mollica, R. F. (1976), Overview: Ethical issues in contemporary psychiatry. *Am. J. Psychiatry* 133:125–136.

Rettig, R. A. (1976), The policy debate on patient care financing for victims of end-stage renal disease. *Law and Contemporary Problems* 40(4): 196–230.

Roberts, C. A., ed. (1968), *Primary Prevention of Psychiatric Disorder*. Toronto: University of Toronto Press.

Rockefeller, N. (1972), Message to the New York State Legislature, January 30, 1972. Reprinted in New York State Planning Committee on Mental Disorders (1975), *Plan for a Comprehensive Mental Health and Mental Retardation Program for New York State*, vol. VII, p. 5.

Rutter, M. (1966), *Children of Sick Patients: An Environmental and Psychiatric Study*. London: Oxford University Press.

Schloendorff v. New York Hospital (1914), 211 N.Y. 127, 129, 105 N.E. 92, 93.

Stone, A. A. (1979), Informed consent: Special problems for psychiatry. *Hosp. Community Psychiatry* 30:321–327.

Struening, E. L. (1977), Social epidemiology in the evaluation of clinical services. In: *New Trends of Psychiatry in the Community,* ed. G. Serban. Cambridge, Massachusetts: Ballinger.

Stubblebine, J. M. & Decker, J. B. (1971), Are urban mental health centers worth it? Part II. *Am. J. Psychiatry* 128:480–483.

Tucker, E. (1966), Troublesome cases in community care. *Milbank Mem. Fund Q.* 44 (1, pt. 2):184–193.

Weston, W. D. (1975), Development of community psychiatry concepts. In: *Comprehensive Textbook of Psychiatry/II,* ed. A. M. Freedman et al. Baltimore: Williams and Wilkins, chapter 43, p. 2311.

Williams, G. et al. (1973), Prediction of the burden of relapsed mental patients. *Community Ment. Health J.* 9:303–315.

Chapter 4

Consequences of the Recommendations of the Privacy Protection Study Commission for Longitudinal Studies*

LEE N. ROBINS

Importance of Identifiable Records for Longitudinal Research

Records are useful to many kinds of social research, but to the longitudinal study, their availability in individually identifiable form is crucial. Longitudinal studies use such records for four main purposes: sampling, locating subjects for interview and locating additional records about them, verifying interview data, and obtaining data for its own sake.

With respect to sampling, access to pertinent records allows choosing the sample from rosters established before the outcome of interest could have occurred. The great advantage of choosing samples from records created before the period of risk is that such samples are unbiased with respect to that outcome —that is, the outcome cannot have affected the chances of an individual's appearance in the sample. This is not true of samples selected during or after the period of risk, for example, in household surveys of adults. Records such as birth records, school records, armed service records, selective service records, and records of children's clinics afford access to appropriate samples of the general population or populations with special problems. If virtually complete recovery of the selected samples is achieved at follow-up, an unbiased sample is achieved.

Identifiable records also are helpful in follow-up studies for lo-

*Reprinted from *Origins of Psychopathology,* edited by Ricks and Dohrenwend and used by permission of Cambridge University Press.

cating individuals for interview, and identifiers found in one set of records help to locate other records. Records may provide current addresses or contain names and addresses of employers or relatives who know current addresses. Further, new addresses found in a record file that includes complete identifiers, such as birth date or social security number, may make it possible to positively identify a research subject in other records that lack complete identifiers.

The use of records to verify information obtained by interview may be particularly important when the outcome variables of interest are likely to be concealed in interview because they are considered disgraceful or perhaps do not redound to the credit of the individual being interviewed. Access to records that enable confirmation or refutation of reported information does not only test the respondents' veracity with respect to verifiable items but, when verifiable discreditable information is found to be freely acknowledged, it may also enhance confidence in the accuracy of other items that cannot be directly verified.

Records are also important sources of outcome data not obtainable by interview alone. Some data of interest may be unknown to the subject, for example, a physician's diagnosis of anxiety neurosis that was recorded but not revealed to the subject. Similarly, it is not possible to learn from a parent who gave a child up for adoption how well the child succeeded in school if the parent has lost contact with the adopted child; school records can provide that information. Further, data in records may be more accurate than data reported by a respondent, no matter how willingly. For instance, if research requires knowing whether truancy typically predates or postdates the first juvenile arrest, a respondent may be able to recall both truancy and arrest but be unable to remember which came first.

Records may have an advantage over interviews, even when information is equally available from either source, becuse record searches avoid invading privacy or interfering with the subject's personal life. One can, for instance, learn from local police records whether an individual has ever been arrested during the follow-up interval. If that is the only outcome of interest, it will not be necessary to recontact the subject for a second interview. Similarly, if the outcome of concern is the school achievement of the index subject's adult offspring, school records can provide that information without involving anyone who had not participated in the initial phase of the study and may not be motivated to participate as a secondary subject.

Finally, data available from records are protected against bias on the part of both subject and interviewer. For example, interviews investigating the transmission of behavior between generations may tend to exaggerate similarities between parent and child because either the respondent or the interviewer believes that behavior in parents often forecasts the same behavior in the child. Such bias is avoided when information on parent and child behavior is obtained from independently constructed records, i.e., records made by separate persons who had no knowledge of the existence of the other records.

For all six reasons—improved sampling, easier location, verification of interviews, provision of otherwise unavailable data, avoidance of unnecessary intrusion into the lives of subjects and their families, and avoidance of biased information —personally identifiable records can play an important role in follow-up studies. However, since the passage in 1974 of the Privacy Act and the Educational Rights Act, access to records without permissions obtained directly from subjects has become very difficult and often illegal. These laws were designed not with research in mind but to assure that record information could not be used against persons without their knowledge, a commendable goal; their effect on longitudinal research is a largely unforeseen side effect. The laws unfortunately failed to distinguish between the use of records for research and statistical purposes and their use for administrative or clinical reasons.

Privacy Protection Study Commission

The Privacy Protection Study Commission was set up by Congress in 1975 to review the whole question of federal regulation with respect to privacy. The Commission's main goal was not to discuss the problems existing laws created for research enterprises, but the Commission did indeed recognize such problems and devoted a chapter to these issues in their Report (Privacy, 1977). In preparation for writing the report, the Commission heard more than 300 witnesses and received many written statements (including one from me). The Report represented the

Commission's efforts to resolve tensions between those who felt it was important that researchers have access to records and those who did not. The Commission made excellent suggestions for repairing some of the damage done by the 1974 laws. One of their most important contributions was to underscore the vital distinction between administrative use of records and statistical and research use. Administrative use was defined as use that is interested in and can have consequences for the subject as an individual. Statistical and research use is interested in the subject only as a representative of a class of individuals and assures that any information collected will not affect the subject as an individual.

My purpose here is to comment on the Report of the Privacy Protection Study Commission and its recommendations as they affect access to personally identifiable records in longitudinal research. As pointed out above, the essence of longitudinal research is the linking of information about individuals that is collected independently at two or more different times. Those who disapprove allowing researchers access to personally identifiable records have argued that one can make do by studying a population longitudinally without individual links. There is ample evidence that this is not the case. To take one example, turnover tables of alcohol abuse show that the *overall level* of problem drinking in the population is quite constant over time, but that *different* people are problem drinkers at different times. The knowledge only of rates of alcoholism in the population as a whole does not reveal what makes for remission or for late onset.

While the recommendations of the Commission would certainly improve access to records for longitudinal research, they would not by any means solve all the problems. I will argue for specific revisions of the Commission's recommendations that I think would again make it possible to do excellent longitudinal research without breaching confidentiality. A breach of confidentiality, I believe, is the only threat to research subjects from most longitudinal studies. My assertion that a breach of confidentiality can be avoided even when access to individually identifiable records is allowed applies to research that selects its sample from a large population and is conducted by persons with no administrative responsibility for members of that sample. The problems of research on small populations, such as one town or the U.S. Congress, and of in-house research by a treatment agency are ticklish ones with respect to confidentiality, whether the research is longitudinal or cross-sectional. When the population is small or made up of well-known people, it becomes virtually impossible to hide identities. If the research is in-house, the research subject cannot easily be convinced that information told to the interviewer can never be obtained by someone with responsibility for making decisions about the subject's future. What I am addressing, then, is the easiest case in which to preserve confidentiality, that is, the collection of information over time about sample members from a large population by an academic or commercial research team that has no connection with or responsibility for any actions concerning the subjects' future.

The Commission noted that longitudinal research entails a greater risk of breach of confidentiality than does cross-sectional research:

The Commission recognizes that identifiers must be retained in some kinds of research, most notably longitudinal and panel survey studies which refer to the same respondents from time to time, but retention should be the exception, not the rule. The decision to retain identifiers should not be left solely to the discretion of researchers. . . . Furthermore, the retention of identifiers should trigger special precautions, such as maintaining face-sheet information separate from the survey instrument, or recording personal identifiers in a separate file that is cross-referenced to the rest of the data [p. 584].

I would agree that maintaining confidentiality in longitudinal studies encounters special problems, but it is important to recognize that the precautions outlined in the quoted paragraph and other available techniques have successfully maintained confidentiality of files kept for many years.

Aside from the dangers of breach of confidentiality, the Privacy Commission dealt with one other type of threat, oversurveying, particularly in captive populations such as school children. This is a legitimate concern for certain populations, but for noncaptive populations, or research using unobtrusive techniques such as record reviews, oversurveying does not seem to be a problem, particularly given the current low funding levels for research. The chance that a member of the general public will be oversurveyed seems rather remote at present.

Comments on Six Commission Recommendations

I would like to discuss six of the Commission's recommendations. These concerned which records are to be available to research, when permissions should expire, the principle of limited disclosure, agency responsibility for judging the merit of research, restrictions on redisclosure, and prompt destruction of identifiers in research records.

Selective Opening of Records

First, the Commission recommended opening certain agency records to research without requiring individually signed permission forms. These include medical records, school records, records of most federal agencies except those now restricted by law, and records of social agencies. The argument in favor of opening medical records stated:

Although a researcher's obligation to obtain an individual's informed consent to participate in any study that may expose him to physical or psychological harm is widely recognized, the researcher's obligation to obtain the patient's permission to use information in records about him has always seemed less compelling. For one thing, the practical difficulties are considerable. Patients are difficult to locate, and if asked for an authorization might refuse, thereby skewing the results of the study in unknown ways. Insistence on patient authorization would make many important studies impossible. The recent search for the cause of the "Legionnaires' Disease," for example, would have been doomed at the start if the researchers had had to obtain authorizations before reviewing medical records [p. 309].

While research would certainly benefit from having the records listed by the Commission reopened to research without requiring individual permissions, the Commission did not suggest freeing other records of great research value and came out strongly in favor of restricting access to some of them, for example, credit and employment records. The Commission apparently did not recognize the role these records can play in health research.

The Commission also failed to recognize that the Government's interest in health, which is presented as a major reason for opening medical records, applies not only after a disorder comes to treatment and appears in a medical record but also to indicators of risk for morbidity and mortality, indicators that play an important role in preventive medicine. Simultaneous appearance in some combination of police records, poor credit ratings, applications for unemployment compensation, poor work attendance records, and records of discipline problems in the military is an excellent early indicator of alcoholism and drug abuse and thus prognosticates the associated physical illnesses of tuberculosis, pneumonia, cirrhosis, hepatitis, and cancers of the mouth, esophagus, and cervix. These records can also serve as excellent measures of treatment effectiveness, much better measures for some disorders than return visits to a physician. If drug treatment is followed by no further arrest, no unemployment or absenteeism, and no failure to pay back loans, this is much better evidence of "success" than is the absence of morphine in the urine.

Unfortunately, rather than recognizing the usefulness of police, credit, and employment records for research purposes, the Commission applauded the narrowest definition of access to credit and employment records:

That the Federal Fair Credit Reporting Act be amended to provide that information concerning an individual maintained by a credit bureau may be used only for credit-related purposes, unless otherwise directed or authorized by the individual [p. 87].

That each employer be considered to owe a duty of confidentiality to any individual employee . . . and that, therefore, no employer or consumer-reporting agency . . . should disclose, or be required to disclose, in individually identifiable form, any information about any individual applicant, employee, or former employee, without the explicit authorization of such individuals, unless the disclosure would be:

(a) In response to a request to provide or verify information designated by the employer as directory information, which should not include more than:
    (i)   the fact of past or present employment;
    (ii)   dates of employment;
    (iii)   title or position;
    (iv)   wage or salary; and
    (v)   location of job site;

(b) an individual's dates of attendance at work and home address in response to a request by a properly identified law enforcement authority . . . [p. 272].

(The exception in [b], which opens attendance records only to a law enforcement agency, was apparently intended to allow presence at work to serve as an alibi for an employee accused of a crime.)

I would like to see the recommendation of access to medical (p. 306), school (p. 441), social agency (p. 476), and federal agency (p. 602) records for research purposes generalized to include *all* records when the appropriate provisions for confidentiality are met. Not only credit and employment records would then become available but also those government agency records which by law or regulation may not now be disclosed in individually identifiable form: records of the Census, Social Security, and Internal Revenue Service. These records would be valuable research resources for longitudinal studies.

Expiration Dates

The Commission recommended that permissions obtained from individuals for access to record information about them remain effective for as brief a period as possible. As one example, the Commission recommended that the duration of permission granted an employer to obtain record information about a prospective employee should not exceed one year. The impact of such restricted permission periods on longitudinal research was not discussed.

If authorizations obtained by researchers remain in effect for so brief a period, it becomes extremely difficult to carry out longitudinal research. The only recourse for a researcher engaged in a follow-up covering several years is a yearly up-date of subject permissions, leading to both unnecessary intrusion into subjects' lives and the risk of altering the representativeness of a sample if some subjects resent the repeated imposition and refuse. If the subjects are willing to grant permissions for longer periods, why should they not be allowed to do so? I would like to see an exemption for longitudinal research in the recommendation for early expiration dates of permissions.

Limited Disclosure

The Commission recommended: That any disclosure of medical-record information by a medical-care provider, with or without the authorization of the individual to whom it pertains, be limited only to information necessary to accomplish the purpose for which the disclosure is made [p. 313].

If this recommendation were accepted literally, it would create havoc in all record research enterprises. The researcher never needs *all* the information in any medical record, for instance. A strict interpretation would mean that the staff of a medical facility would have to abstract medical records for the researcher to keep the researcher from seeing unneeded material. This would severely reduce the quality of the data collected, since the clerk so assigned by the agency would be both uninterested in the research project and untrained for the purpose. Also, it would mean that medical records would seldom be available to research, since few medical agencies would have staff with sufficient time to do the abstracting. My suggestion would be to simply state that the agency should be permitted to disclose only those records that contain information necessary to the research.

Agency Judgment of the Merit of the Research

One of the Committee's conditions for opening records for research and statistical purposes without the consent of the concerned individuals is expressed in Guideline 3(c) and repeated with respect to each type of record for which disclosure is recommended. This provision states that the entity (i.e., the agency that has control over the records):

determines that the research or statistical purpose for which any disclosure is to be made is of sufficient social benefit to warrant the increase in the risk to the individual of exposure of the record or information [p. 602].

To fulfill this requirement, the government agency holding the record would have to decide on the scientific merit of the research. Clearly, poorly designed research is of no social benefit. However, this requirement seems excessive, since research projects for which records are sought will often be supported by federal grants and thus have been judged to have scientific merit by the peer review process. I have heard informally that the National Institute of Mental Health (NIMH) has already decided to accept grant approval as evidence of merit rather than ask the record-holding agency to make this decision. It seems to me that it ought to be official rather than unofficial policy that a federally funded project shall be considered of sufficient social benefit to merit the release of information from records. The necessity for formalizing this policy becomes clear when one realizes that research projects often need to link information from various agencies. If only one agency decides it is unable to judge the scientific merit of the project, its refusal to grant access to its records may compromise a whole project.

My suggestion is that Guideline 3(c) read:

. . . determines that the research has met tests of feasibility, scientific soundness, and ethical standards through peer review and institutional review procedures.

Restrictions on Redisclosure

According to the Commission Report's Guideline 3(e), (and repeated elsewhere in the Report), in addition to judging a research proposal's merit, the agency in control of records:

prohibits any further use or redisclosure of the record or information in individually identifiable form without its express authorization [p. 602].

Enacting this recommendation would mean that once records had been obtained and the follow-up completed, no future follow-up would be possible without again getting permission from the same agency. This raises two important issues.

First, a decision to do a second follow-up study might be made as much as fifteen to twenty years after the original study. Examples of follow-up studies repeated long after the end of the initially planned final data collection can be found in Vaillant's (1977) reopening of the Grant study, McCord's (1978) refollow-up of the Cambridge-Somerville study, and Block's (1971) continuation of the Berkeley Guidance and Oakland Growth Study follow-ups. During such long intervals, the agency that provides the original records may well become reorganized, making it difficult to find an authority to give permission for further use of the records.

Second, in the course of a follow-up study that begins with records obtained from a government agency, the researcher amplifies the identifiers obtained from agency records. Telephone numbers may be added, addresses updated, relatives listed who can help to locate subjects. Why should the government agency that provided the original records have the right to prevent the use at some future date of data the researcher created during the study? Thus, the restriction seems unenforceable as well as undesirable.

Rather than requiring a return to the original agency for permission to do a second follow-up, I recommend that Guideline 3(e) be revised to state:

. . . prohibits further use or redisclosure unless the further use is for research that conforms to all the rules set for preserving confidentiality of the data and meets tests of feasibility, scientific soundness, and ethical standards as specified for the original study.

This recommendation would ensure that standards applied in the first research use of the records apply in all subsequent use.

Destruction of Records

The Commission strongly recommended that the identifiers on research records be destroyed as soon as the research is completed:

The Commission believes that the single most important procedure for maintaining the confidentiality of research and statistical data is the prompt removal and destruction of identifiers . . . ideally, identifiers should be removed or destroyed as soon as the data are collected and verified [p. 584].

If an application is for school records, Recommendation 4(c) further specifies:

that records created about an unsuccessful applicant be maintained by an educational agency or institution for 18 months after the close of the application process, after which time they must be destroyed [p. 434].

If these recommendations were followed, no cross-sectional study could become the basis for a later follow-up unless the follow-up had been planned from the beginning. This would be a tragedy. One simply cannot predict ahead of time when it may be of great social value to follow up subjects from an earlier study. The discovery of the delayed adverse outcomes of exposure to radiation and to the hormone DES during pregnancy are among the many examples that come to mind. There was no way of anticipating decades earlier that identifiers for subjects in various drug trials should be saved for later follow-up.

The Census saves its records for 72 years in the National Archives, at which point the records enter the public domain. While I do not suggest that all research records go to the National Archives, various methods can be used to keep identifiers safely separate from research protocols for many years. A key linking the two can be maintained in a safety deposit box, for instance, so that the two coud be reunited in the future if necessary for a longitudinal study. The destruction of identifiers precludes that opportunity forever. I would like to delete the Commission's recommendations for destruction of identifiers and substitute the requirement that identifiers be kept separate from research protocols and secured in such a way that the two cannot be linked without permission from the principal investigator or a designated agent.

Suggestions to Make Recommended Revisions More Acceptable

All the suggestions I have made so far liberalize researchers' access to records. Perhaps some new restrictions also should be added. One of the reasons the Commission is uneasy about researchers' use of data is that confidentiality has been violated in the past by inadequately trained researchers. The Report describes a case reported to the Commission:

. . . a researcher was doing a follow-up study of people who had been enrolled in a methadone maintenance program . . . the contractor had the name and address of one particular individual who had been enrolled in the program several years previously, and the contractor went to the individual's residence. It was Saturday night, and the person was having a party and the contractor said, "Hi, I am so-and-so from such-and-such an organization, and we are doing a follow-up study of patients who have been enrolled in the methadone maintenance program" [p. 309].

Clearly, such behavior is reprehensible, and competent researchers do not act that way. However, it is notable that regulations aimed at preserving confidentiality have been addressed more often to protecting research records than to data collection. I know of no formal code designed to minimize the risks of breach of confidentiality during the data collection period. The following items, which have appeared in a manual for use in following drug patients (Robins & Smith, 1977), might be included in such a code:

(1) In case-control studies, that is, studies in which affected and non-affected individuals are selected for follow-up, the identity of the individual as case or control must be separated from other identifiers during the period of data collection, so that there will be no disclosure of the case or control status to agencies from which information is being sought, in case those agencies might have administrative interest in the subjects, or to subjects' relatives or acquaintances from whom help in locating him might be sought.

(2) If no control subjects, i.e., no subjects with "nonincriminating" identities, are to be included in the study, lists of subjects must be liberally salted with random names before submitting them to agencies for acquisition of data or locating information, so that agencies from which further data are sought will have no assurance that any particular individual on the list is of administrative interest to them.

(3) When record information other than identifiers is obtained prior to interviewing subjects, interviewers must be kept ignorant of that record information so that there will be no danger of their disclosing such information to the subject or to anyone else.

(4) Research studies on sensitive topics should be required to develop an innocuous description of the study and innocuous letterheads for contacting employers or relatives for help in locating subjects, so that mere participation as a study subject does not in itself give away any information that interested parties might not already have.

Following these strictures would prevent the kinds of unfortunate disclosures during collection of research data described in the examples presented to the Commission. Once data are collected, separation of identifiers from protocols maintains confidentiality. The only remaining danger of disclosure then lies with the government itself through the power of the courts.

The Commission advocated protection of research records from subpoena:

The Commission has concluded that the individual's privacy interests as well as his right to refuse to testify against himself demand, albeit indirectly, that research and statistical records be generally immune to disclosure compelled by judicial order . . . [p. 579].

The Commission did not, however, recommend total immunity, but would allow disclosure in court if necessary to prosecute a researcher or research institution for violating the law. These seem reasonable limitations.

Until such time as there are laws exempting research records from subpoena, researchers are in a very difficult position. If a researcher has guaranteed confidentiality to a respondent, it seems to me that this amounts to a promise to destroy lists of identifiers in the face of a subpoena, even if it means having to go to jail. In my and my colleagues' research with veterans, we have hoped to avoid this risk by keeping the list pairing name identification numbers with protocol identification numbers outside the borders of the United States, so that the only remaining danger period is while the interview is still in the hands of the interviewer. We have told our interviewers we expect them to honor their obligation to destroy the identifiers or the protocol should the interview be demanded by law enforcement officers before it has been mailed. Since none of us wants to go to jail, and since maintaining a "foreign connection" is onerous, I recommend immunity of research records from subpoena.

Finally, the problem of risks and benefits should be examined from the point of view of the agencies whose cooperation is necessary to obtain records for longitudinal research. So far, the focus has been exclusively on the needs of research subjects. Risks to the agency administration may be at least as great, and the agency usually has nothing to gain from letting its records be used in a research enterprise. One federal agency to whose records I and my colleagues needed access asked the Department of Justice for an opinion as to whether the records could legally be given to us. When this assurance of legality was obtained, the head of the agency was still uneasy and said, "I know now that I *can* let you have the records. But I *can* go out and stand in traffic, too."

We are grateful to that agency head for having decided to let us have the records despite his feeling that he was taking grave risks, that is, "standing in traffic." But the example indicates that there should be rewards for the agency that collaborates in research, benefits that better balance the risks. Those of us who do longitudinal research need the help of agencies that collect the records we use. We need to reduce the risks and increase the agencies' rewards for helping us.

Acknowledgments

This work was supported by U.S. Public Health Service grants DA 00013, MH 18894, and AA 03539. It is a revised and updated version of a chapter in *Origins of Psychopathology* (1983), ed. D. F. Ricks & B. S. Dohrenwend. Cambridge, England: Cambridge University Press.

References

Block, J. (1971), *Lives Through Time*. Berkeley: Bancroft Books.

McCord, J. (1978), A thirty-year follow-up of treatment effects. *Am. Psychologist* 33 (3):284–298.

Privacy Protection Study Commission Report (1977), *Personal Privacy in an Information Society*. Washington, D.C.: U.S. Government Printing Office.

Robins, L. & Smith, J. E. (1977), Ethical considerations and confidentiality. In: *Conducting Follow-Up Research on Drug Treatment Programs;* ed. L. Johnston, D. N. Nurco, & L. N. Robins. Treatment Program Monograph Series Number 2, National Institute on Drug Abuse.

Vaillant, G. (1977), *Adaptation to Life*. Boston: Little, Brown.

Chapter 5

Ethics and Public Policy in High-Risk Research

NATALIE ABRAMS

There is strong evidence that children of schizophrenics have a greater likelihood than the average person of becoming schizophrenic. The question, therefore, frequently arises as to how the important genetic and familial factors involved in the transmission of mental illness can best be researched without creating serious emotional distress for high-risk participants. Should children of a schizophrenic parent, for example, be informed of their high risk of developing this condition? Some researchers may argue against the conveying of such information, pointing out their potential detrimental psychological effects. On the other hand, informing high-risk subjects of their vulnerable position may work to their benefit. This was brought out poignantly in a piece written by a Haverford senior named A. L. Sandridge for the *Bryn Mawr Alumni Bulletin* (Winter 1984:19) in which she discussed her mother's mental illness and "genetic predisposition to schizophrenia" and her own research interests in studying the factors that may be responsible for mental illness in women, such as the impact of the mental health care system itself. She went on to state that even though she has "probably the same genetic disposition as her mother," nevertheless, she "will probably escape schizophrenia" primarily because the accepting and supportive environment in which she has grown up has allowed her a wider range of behaviors than has been customary for women during earlier periods.

This paper is a discussion of some ethical and public policy issues presented by prospective studies of the transmission of mental illness, frequently referred to as follow-up high-risk research. The first section briefly describes this type of research; the second section relates the research to several ethical principles underlying our society's research guidelines; and the third section discusses some public policy issues that emerge from the research.

Features of High-Risk Research

The goal of high-risk research is to discover what predisposing factors place certain individuals at risk for becoming mentally ill. To date, most such research has focused on the transmission of schizophrenia, and the underlying question concerns the respective roles of environment versus heredity in the development of the disease (Kimling, 1979). Great confusion over this issue results from different formulations of the question (Rosenthal, 1968).

One common formulation asks whether schizophrenia is inherited. Evidence shows clearly that in any strict sense schizophrenia is not simply an inherited disease, since not everyone who possesses the suspected genotype becomes schizophrenic. Furthermore, studies of monozygotic twins indicate that one twin may develop the disease and the other may not. These facts have led some to be skeptical about the role of heredity. A second formulation asks whether schizophrenia is inherited in the sense that any individual with the involved gene(s) is either "basically or potentially" schizophrenic, even without clinical manifestations. However, this question is empirically unanswerable. A third formulation asks whether the development of schizophrenia depends partly on having the requisite genotype but more importantly on environmental factors. If so, the clinical manifestation of schizophrenia would result from the interaction of a particular genotype with particular life experiences. In this view, schizophrenia is generally thought not to be an inherited disorder. The underlying question has been phrased by Erlenmeyer-Kimling: "What kinds of environmental input trigger manifestations of the disorder in genotypically vulnerable persons, and why are these important in a psycho-physiological sense?" (Rosenthal, 1968).

High-risk research aims at identifying both the genetic and environmental factors implicated in the development of schizophrenia. Such research can take two different forms. On the one hand, there can be cross-sectional studies, which are essentially retrospective. In such studies, parents of children who suffer from schizophrenia or other behavioral disorders are questioned about their children's development and previous history. Numerous difficulties with such studies have been elaborated by Robins (1970): first, the parents might interpret rather than simply report past experiences in order to explain the child's present behavior; second, in an attempt to explain the child's problem, such parents might recall and place significance on past incidents which other parents would not even remember; third, such parents might not be able to take a realistic view of their own behavior as parents and consequently either exaggerate or fail to recognize their own personal mode of interaction; and fourth, as any parent might do, parents of disturbed children might simply recall situations incorrectly.

On the other hand, the research methodology for discovering individuals at high-risk may take the form of follow-up studies, which are essentially prospective. In such studies, normal children are followed over a number of years to determine what influences do or do not produce mental illness. In most such studies, a group of normal children of schizophrenic parent(s) are followed concomitantly with a control group of normal children of parent(s) with no history of mental disturbance. As much as possible the two groups are matched for numerous variables, such as age, sex, and economic and social class. Designing follow-up studies in such a way attempts to obviate some of the problems of cross-sectional research in that the accumulation of data does not depend on memory with all of its possible distortions. The main advantages of follow-up studies are said to be: "1) that information about early life is more accurate; 2) the temporal order between environmental factors and the development of psychiatric disorder can sometimes be ascertained; and 3) a more complete sample of the population can be achieved" (Robins, 1970).

Robins further identifies two different types of follow-up studies. One type follows children from birth through some specified age, supposedly the termination of childhood, and determines how many develop problems during that period. A second type follows normal children of various ages for a fixed period of time, long enough so that some of them will have reached the end of childhood, and determines how many cases of disorders appear. The Berkeley Growth Study (Macfarlane et al., 1954) exemplifies the first method, and two Swedish studies, by Jonsson and Kalvesten (Jonsson, 1967), exemplify the second method. In these studies various factors were evaluated as possible indices of behavioral disorders, including socioeconomic factors, parental performance, psychiatric illness in parents, children's early behavior, and traumatic experiences in early childhood.

With regard to schizophrenia, one variable considered particularly significant for the development of the disease is having a schizophrenic parent(s). One of the earliest research models focusing on this factor was that proposed by Pearson & Kley (1957), in which they recommended a longitudinal investigation of children of schizophrenic parents. Other studies prompted by this work, e.g., those by D. Sobel, F. Kallmann, and S. Mednick and F. Schulsinger, were described in an interesting article in *Psychiatric Annals* (Erlenmeyer-Kimling et al., 1979). A primary goal of such studies was to distinguish three different high-risk groups: those without the implicated genotypes; those who are genetically predisposed and do develop the disease; and those who are genetically predisposed who never develop schizophrenia.

Although it is not the purpose of this paper to describe these studies in detail, some information about the general methodology employed is necessary for evaluating the ethical and public policy implications. The study reported by Erlenmeyer-Kimling et al., 1979) included 205 children between the ages of seven and twelve, and the siblings of these "study children" also were followed, although not extensively. Of the study children, 80 were designated high risk, i.e., with a schizophrenic parent(s), and 125 as low risk. Of the low-risk group, 100 had parents who had never been hospitalized for schizophrenia or treated for a psychiatric disorder before the start of the study, and 25 had parents with some other psychiatric disorder not related to schizophrenia. The control group was obtained through volunteers contacted by two large school systems, and the study and control children were matched as much as possible. Intensive interviews were initially conducted in the subjects' homes, followed by a full day of laboratory testing of the study children. Two-year intervals were planned between each round of testing, during which time the families were contacted by phone at approximately 3–6 month intervals. Additional data included school records, teachers' evaluations, and tests of blood samples.

An alternative methodology was employed in a study by Sobel (1961) in which a group of newborn infants with two schizophrenic parents were followed from birth. The goal was to record direct observations of how such parents cared for and interacted with their infants. Immediately following birth, the infants were observed in the nursery. Subsequently, half went to live with foster parents and the other half went home to their schizophrenic parents. Monthly home observations were made, lasting approximately 1–3 hours. Attempts were made not to disrupt normal routine and yet to be present at significant times of interaction, e.g., during feeding or bathing. Obviously, one of the goals was to compare the interactions and follow-up behavior of the children who went home to their natural parents with those who went to live with foster parents.

The work of Heston (1966) suggests another approach to studying the transmission of schizophrenia. Heston studied adults born to schizophrenic mothers but separated from their natural mothers immediately following birth, who never lived with any maternal relatives. Some went to live with paternal relatives, others were placed in foundling homes. Comparisons were made with a control group from the same foundling homes who were matched for sex, type of eventual placement (adoptive, foster family, or institutional), and for length of time in child-care institutions. Assessments of the individuals' psychosocial adjustment were subsequently based upon school, police, veterans, and hospital records, as well as on personal interviews and psychiatric evaluations.

Crossfostering is another technique employed to help solve the environment-heredity controversy. This strategy involves studying adopted-away offspring of normal biological parents who are reared by schizophrenic parents. Comparisons are made between this group and adopted-away offspring of schizophrenic biological parents reared by normal adopting parents and adopted-away offspring of normal biological parents reared by normal adopting parents. In such a study conducted in Denmark (Wender et al., 1974) the subjects underwent intensive psychiatric interviews and a day and a half of psychological tests. Adoptees did not know their biological heritage or the psychiatric status of their biological parents.

From the above, it is evident that a variety of research methodologies are employed in high-risk research. In some, children of a schizophrenic parent(s) are followed and compared with children of normal parents. Both sets are raised by their biological parents. In other studies, adopted-away offspring of both normal and schizophrenic parents are compared when reared by either normal or schizophrenic adoptive parents. Some studies follow children from birth, others make the initial contact during the crucial age range of seven to twelve, and others compare adults born to schizophrenic parents (separated from the biological parents at birth) with adults born to normal parents.

Implicit in all these methodologies is an important problem that should not be overlooked, difficulties in the case identification essential to any epidemiological research. The problem has two aspects: first, the difficulty of defining the mental disorder under consideration, in this case schizophrenia; second, the difficulty of identifying the disorder in a given individual to be sure that a subject actually manifests the disease. Without shared diagnostic categories and validated case identifications, much epidemiological research, including high-risk research, becomes meaningless.

An additional dimension to this problem arises with regard to the classification of childhood disorders. As pointed out by Robins (1970), since psychiatric diagnosis relies heavily on past history, and a child patient had such a short past and so little history, diagnosis and prognosis of the illness in a child are extremely difficult. Furthermore, attempts to use so-called more objective criteria than history in case identification present new difficulties. The fact of hospitalization or a previous physician's diagnosis may reflect cultural influences rather than the confirmed existence of mental illness. These problems, as well as many others, e.g., distinguishing between a truly increased incidence rate and merely an increase in the reporting of a disease, must therefore be kept in mind when evaluating data accumulated in psychiatric epidemiology. Although the goal of high-risk research is worthwhile, namely "intervention in order to prevent the development of schizophrenic disorder" (Kimling et al., 1979) in view of these difficulties great caution would seem to be warranted before using such data to plan any intervention programs.

Ethical Issues

Ethical issues are raised by at least two distinct aspects of high-risk research: the research methodologies themselves and the possible information to be gained. Four basic principles underlying our society's research guidelines are called into question by both aspects: the principle of autonomy, or individual consent; the principle of acceptable level of risk; the principle of privacy; and the principle of liberty.

Autonomy/Consent

Autonomy is essentially the right to self-determination, as formulated in the Declaration of Independence. Individuals are the bearers of rights they cannot give away or sell, which can be abridged only with their consent. One is that of self-determination, which in the medical context becomes the right to decide what shall happen with or to one's own body. Whereas the requirement of informed consent might be overridden by the physician's therapeutic privilege in certain situations, it becomes significantly stricter in a nontherapeutic research context. Given the fact that high-risk research is primarily nontherapeutic, it entails a very stringent demand to obtain as full a consent as possible. Interviews with parents pose no special difficulties, but complications arise when they give consent not only on their own behalf but on behalf of their children—traditionally referred to as "proxy consent" and, more recently, as "substituted judgment."

Assuming that the right to consent allows one to decide exactly as one wishes, regardless of the opinion of others, and that one person can therefore not truly "consent" for another, the difficult question concerns the basis upon which substituted judgment should be accepted. In some situations, e.g., those involving young children, of necessity true consent is not possible. Alternative criteria have been suggested as the basis for substituted judgment, for example, to try to act toward the "voiceless" as we would ordinarily act toward competent adults, i.e., to decide as the individual (the child, or incompetent adult) would decide if capable. This is known as the hypothetical test, which seems feasible with previously able but now incompetent adults. In situations concerning the termination of treatment in such cases, family members or a living will can give evidence of an adult patient's wishes. With children, however, the situation is considerably more problematic, both logically and practically. Should the "proxy" try to decide as an adult looking back to the proxy's own childhood, or as a selfless, objective surrogate guessing from intimate knowledge what the child subject would most likely want? It might be almost impossible for the proxy to refrain from substituting personal wishes for those of the child.

A second criterion sometimes suggested for substituted judgment is to attempt to decide as the individual *should* decide, on the basis of the concept of social obligation. According to this view, we are all beneficiaries of research conducted on other people and therefore also have an obligation to participate. Furthermore, the argument is sometimes made that when the risk is minimal, the consent of children for nontherapeutic research may be presumed since such research is frequently the only means by which information can be gained to benefit a whole population. Certainly, it is not always possible to generalize to children from research conducted on adults, whether it involves drug effectiveness or toxicity or the precursors to schizophrenia; children are not miniature adults. An important implication of this suggested criterion should be noted. In deciding as an individual should decide, additional considerations are usually included, such as the interests of parents, siblings, society, or even the health care professionals. Included in the decision-making process, therefore, are concerns traditionally excluded by the concept of personal medical care. This criterion therefore seems unacceptable. Since the consent of adults is not presumed simply because in some sense adults should participate, it does not seem legitimate to presume the consent of children.

A third criterion for substituted judgment is the so-called reasonable man standard. According to this, in the absence of evidence to the contrary it is legitimate to presume that the individual in question, if competent, would act as a reasonable person. Obviously, this presents many difficulties. First, how is one to decide how a reasonable person would act? Second, since a reasonable person is generally considered to be one of the majority, such classification may violate the individual's autonomy to be one of the minority and have idiosyncrasies and peculiarities. Third, since a reasonable member of the majority is generally presumed to choose in his or her best interest, this third criterion actually reduces to a fourth, that of best interest.

According to the best-interest standard, the only legitimate basis upon which one person should decide for another is that of the latter's best interest. Given the difficulties with the other criteria, especially as applied to children, and the fact that in caring for adults only their wishes or possibly best interests are considered, best interest would seem to be the only acceptable standard. In any given situation, the difficult question is then deciding what is in fact in the child's best interest.

Level of Risk

Various features of high-risk research involving children pose the question of whether or not it can be said to be in the child's best interest. First, the research is clearly nontherapeutic, in that the goal is not primarily to benefit the individuals being studied but eventually to gather enough information for future benefit to others. This fact is intimately related to the principle of acceptable level of risk. Surely, when no benefit is to be gained by the research subject, there is a more stringent requirement that the risks be minimal.

What possible risks of harm are in fact incurred by prospective high-risk research, and are they acceptable? This question requires a brief digression concerning the definition of harm itself. One definition of harm is the contravention of an individual's desires or wants. This definition appears excessively broad. On the one hand, many people desire things that are, in the ordinary sense, thought "harmful" to them. On the other hand, many do not desire things ordinarily considered necessary or simply beneficial.

A second definition of harm is the contravention not simply of desires but of an individual's interests. According to this definition, "an object of an interest is what is truly good for a person whether he desires it or not" (Feinberg, 1973). As Feinberg pointed out, however, it is extremely difficult to argue that something undesired is in an individual's interest unless one can show that it would in the long run contribute toward realizing what the individual does desire.

A third definition of harm deals with unmet needs. According to this, an individual is harmed only if needs, rather than interests or desires, are not being met. Whereas the unmet-need definition of harm is minimalistic, i.e., an individual is harmed if not kept at a minimal level of need satisfaction, the definition based on contravention of desires or wants is maximalistic, i.e., an individual is harmed simply by having unfulfilled desires. This same distinction is frequently made by referring to unmet needs versus unneeded benefits or goods. Furthermore, in addition to harm related to level of satisfaction, there are also other, and different, types of harms. Physical injuries are the most obvious but not necessarily the most important; temporary mental distress, intellectual impairment, emotional deprivation or turmoil, and psychological impairment certainly all also count as harms.

Returning to the issues at hand, the original question can now be rephrased. What possible risks for different levels and kinds of harm are acceptable in nontherapeutic research on children, and what does this imply for prospective high-risk research? Assuming some degree of paternalism is warranted in dealing with children, defining harm to them as simple invasion of their desires or wants would be insufficient. However, invasion of their interests interpreted as above, i.e., as integrating long-term wants, would be a more acceptable definition. This definition would correlate with the best-interest standard, whereas the minimalist definition of harm in terms of unmet needs would violate the best-interest standard; simply having one's needs met may be less than equal to having one's best interests protected. Harm would be done if a child's long-term interests were violated.

It should be noted that defining harm as the contravention of long-term interests, in accord with the best-interest standard, would not be appropriate for all contexts. Since it implies a very strict and high-level definition of harm, which demands acting in the child's best interest as the only acceptable behavior, such a definition does seem appropriate for nontherapeutic research, from which the child will receive no benefits. In such a context, the best interest of the child, or the highest standard, should be operative. Such a standard would also be appropriate in custody disputes. However, in other contexts, for example, defining child abuse and neglect, the best-interest standard would appear too stringent. Since some other home environment might always be better for the child, the best-interest standard might frequently require the shifting of children from one home to another. Harm defined minimalistically as unmet needs would therefore seem better suited to questions of abuse and neglect (Abrams, 1979).

From the best-interest view of harm, several features of high-risk research pose the question of whether it violates long-term interests and what kinds of long-term interests. Since prospective studies are concerned with the development of disease, the children when first interviewed and tested are all normal. In fact, precautions are taken to rule out individuals who displayed symptoms of behavioral disorders prior to the research. Consequently, one serious issue is whether questioning normal children, especially those whose parents are schizophrenic, could cause the children to become anxious and overly concerned about their future development and perhaps even their present psychological state. This risk is highlighted by the fact that many of the children are interviewed during the pre-adolescent and adolescent periods when normal children are frequently having self-doubts and going through emotional and physiological changes. At such a period, it would not seem to be in their long-term best interest to have psychiatric personnel further question their psychological status, or for them to have the sense that they will be followed throughout the course of their development. Consent from parents would not be sufficient to overcome the objection that such research could psychologically harm the child.

Simply from the viewpoint of research methodology, an additional difficulty pervades all follow-up research. Is it possible that interviewing and questioning, over a period of time, indirectly produce the behavior being studied? In other words, can the research objective become a self-fulfilling prophecy?

One possible way out of this difficulty is simply not to tell the children the purpose of the research, or perhaps even misinform them. Either approach would be unacceptable, for surely a child of ten, eleven, or twelve has a right to know the purpose of activities in which he or she is engaged; truth-telling should be the norm unless there is a compelling paternalistic justification for lying. High-risk research does not qualify as such an exception since considerably more information would have to be known before justifying interventional or therapeutic programs would be formulated.

Further ethical difficulties are posed by high-risk research on adopted-away offspring of schizophrenic parents. If the adopted children know their biological heritage, the problems are the same as those mentioned above. However, if the adopted children do not know their biological background, is it justifiable to keep this information from them and, if it is kept secret, what should the researcher tell the children about the purpose of the interviews and testing? Similar questions can be asked if the children are adopted-away offspring of normal biological parents raised by parents who are schizophrenic. It should be noted that in research cited earlier, no mention was made about consent, either how consent was obtained or what the children were told, nor were possible research risks recognized. The risks were either unconsidered or considered too insignificant to mention. The former possibility seems unlikely and the latter possibility cannot be accepted on face value. Some way should be built into the research methodology to determine whether the research poses risks for young subjects. Also, some attempt should be made to distinguish the effects of research from the effects of underlying pathology.

Research that follows children from infancy entails slightly different problems. The risk is indirectly causing undue anxiety not in the infant but in the parents, which affects the parent-child relationship. The parents, especially with a first child, may fret unnecessarily about both their relations with the infant and the infant's behavior. Such research also singles out both parents and normal children as potentially mentally ill. Although the ultimate goal of such research may be extremely worthwhile, identification as a special candidate for mental illness is still a stigma in our society. Great precautions must be taken to prevent the risks of stigmatization from outweighing those of becoming ill.

Privacy against Unwanted Intrusion

Privacy and confidentiality of information are guaranteed by the Federal Government in a variety of ways. Specifically, in 1974, Congress passed the Privacy Act which "safeguard(s) individual privacy from the misuse of Federal records" and "provide(s) that individuals be granted access to records concerning them which are maintained by Federal agencies." Individuals have the right to determine the uses made of their personal records and to correct false information. Although this act does not specifically cite medical records, it is believed to affect them as well. In addition, confidentiality is protected in the physician-patient relationship by the law of evidentiary privileges. A privileged communication exists between individuals in special relationships, e.g., physician-patient, lawyer-client, psychotherapist-patient. Since the main purpose of this privilege is to encourage the full disclosure of all information necessary for adequate guidance by the physician or lawyer, the privilege does not necessarily apply to subjects of nontherapeutic research. However, confidentiality of information in nontherapeutic research has been protected by research guidelines recommended by the Department of Health, Education and Welfare (now Health and Human Services).

Questions of privacy arise in relation to two aspects of follow-up high-risk research. First, the issue of privacy concerns preliminary information needed to initiate the research, e.g., about adoption proceedings, psychiatric status of the biological parents, hospital admissions of schizophrenic patients, and children's school records. Without such information it would be impossible to locate schizophrenic parents of school-aged children. Obviously, such information cannot be given anonymously or in aggregate form since the researcher must contact individuals to secure their participation. Second, the issue of privacy concerns information gained during the course of the research. For example, if a child or group of children seems to be at risk for developing behavioral problems, becoming delinquent, etc., should this information be available to police, school, or medical authorities?

The common idea of privacy involved here is very general, with unclear boundaries. For example, it includes such things as private information, which cannot be revealed or demanded; a private space (home), which cannot be observed or intruded upon; a private event, which can be attended only by invited individuals; and private property, which cannot be used by others without the owner's permission.

Privacy as Liberty Right

A constitutional right to so-called privacy was established in *Griswold v. Connecticut* (1965). In this case the Supreme Court overruled a Connecticut statute that forbade the use of contraceptives by married couples. The court's argument was that the statute violated a constitutional right to marital privacy, which was seen as exemplifying a more general right to privacy. Such a general right was located in various amendments of the Bill of Rights, considered jointly. The decision in *Roe v. Wade* (1973), overruling a Texas statute forbidding abortion except to save the mother's life, was also based on the right to privacy, in this case located in the Fourteenth Amendment.

The concept of privacy defended by the Supreme Court decisions seems quite different from the ordinary notion of privacy. Whereas the latter primarily focuses on freedom from intrusion, the former is essentially concerned with autonomy in private decisions. "Primarily and principally the new [Supreme Court] Right of Privacy is a zone of prima facie autonomy, of presumptive immunity from regulation, in addition to that established by the first amendment" (Henkin, 1974). It defends not simply a right against unwarranted intrusion but a much broader liberty right, a right to private zones of behavior or conduct.

Questions of privacy as a liberty right are also posed by prospective high-risk research. Here, however, they concern less the research itself than the potential information to be gained from the research. The fundamental issue is what should be the response, if any, to the discovery of such information as schizophrenia being primarily genetic, or primarily a result of environmental influences, or primarily the result of environmental influences acting on those who are genetically at risk. Possible responses might include mandating screening programs, limiting marriage or procreation rights, removing children from potentially injurious home environments, or even requiring sterilization in some cases. Each response might be seen as an invasion of a constitutionally guaranteed right to privacy, in the sense of a liberty right to private zones of behavior. But, since the right to liberty is not absolute, the question becomes whether other interests or rights exist that override the liberty right to privacy. In legal terms, is there a "compelling state interest" that limits the right?

Various principles or reasons can be put forth as possible justifications for limiting an individual's liberty (Feinberg, 1973). Perhaps the most generally acceptable reason is to prevent harm to others. Feinberg distinguishes two different versions of this: the Private Harm Principle, i.e., preventing harm to individual persons, and the Public Harm Principle, i.e., preventing "impairment of institutional practices that are in the public interest." Alternatively, liberty may be limited to prevent harm to

(Legal Paternalism) or to benefit (Extreme Paternalism) the person whose freedom is being restricted. Liberty may also be limited to benefit others (Welfare Principle). For the most part, our society limits liberty only for prevention of harm rather than production of a benefit—quarantine, inoculation, and the military draft being examples.

How might these reasons for overriding the right to privacy apply to information accumulated through follow-up high-risk research? If it is discovered, for example, that environmental influences, especially parental, are primarily responsible for the development of schizophrenia, would this warrant mandating further screening of all families with schizophrenic parents and then providing follow-up counseling or intervention services either to prevent or treat discovered disorders? Since the data about environmental causes would be likely to show an increased risk for families with schizophrenic parents, screening might reveal other families at risk. Also, the data might not rule out the possibility that similar behavioral patterns or modes of parent-child interaction in nonschizophrenic families could produce children with schizophrenia.

Given the prevalence of schizophrenia, the question of limiting the population for screening would arise. One approach might be mandatory screening, since screening is necessary to give parents enough information upon which to make a fully voluntary and rational decision about accepting or rejecting follow-up services once they were developed. A more interventionist approach, however, might mandate not only the screening but the follow-up services, on the basis of preventing serious harm to others, namely the children (Private Harm Principle), or the community at large (Public Harm Principle).

It might also be argued that mandating either screening or intervention programs would undermine the autonomy and functioning of the family as an institution. It might be less deleterious to the children involved, and to society as a whole, to allow the family considerable autonomy and to intervene as little as possible. This reasoning cites the Public Harm Principle to justify nonintervention. Such reasoning was, in fact, employed by Justice Burger in a Supreme Court ruling granting parents the right to place their children in mental institutions, rather than having the state "interfering" with families functioning smoothly on their own.

Another very significant issue must be recognized in connection with screening programs: the possibility of false positives. A family may be incorrectly identified as presenting a risk for the children, thus creating undue anxiety and disturbance as well as the possible risk that the disturbance itself might induce behavioral disorders in the children or adversely affect parent-child interactions.

Limiting procreation or custody rights might also be considered if research strongly supported the conclusion that either genetics or family environment produces schizophrenia. An analogy might be drawn to the situation of child abuse or neglect, in which it is sometimes thought legitimate to remove children from homes in which parents abused or neglected their children or if parents were judged unfit to rear the children. The disruptions of family life by a schizophrenic parent(s) and, in many cases, the repeated placement of children in temporary foster homes may be at least prima facie cause for removal of the children. Limiting procreation rights would be considerably more problematic. What harm to what person would thereby be prevented? Can it ever be said to be better for an individual not to have been born? This has far-reaching implications, since many disturbances or problems, genetic or otherwise, could have been prevented had the individuals simply not been born. Consistency would demand a similar approach to numerous genetic abnormalities.

Similar principles might be applied to justify overriding proscriptions against violating our ordinary notion of privacy. Releasing certain information to school or police authorities might be justified either by the desire to prevent harm to the individual child, to benefit the child, or to prevent harm to society as a whole. For example, information about a child's psychological status may be crucial to educational development.

Ultimately, these questions about consent, level of risk, and privacy are public policy issues. The following is a brief discussion of alternative conceptions of public policy and possible vehicles for resolving some of the issues.

Public Policy Issues

Underlying the problem of formulating public policy responses to the issues discussed above is the question of whether such issues should be considered in the public or private realm. If all decisions about consent, level of risk, sterilization, procreation, the rearing of children, and the release of personal information are necessarily private, then it might appear inappropriate to formulate public policies for them. However, this view is narrow-minded in several ways. First, a considerable precedent in child abuse and neglect legislation, as well as in the *parens patriae* (state as parent in special cases) power of the state, tends to support the view that the public should have a say on such questions. Second, decisions on such issues are not completely self-regarding, in that other individuals are ultimately affected, namely, the children involved as well as society as a whole, in terms of possible future burdens. Decisions that affect others in such significant ways cannot be automatically taken to be private. Third, even if such issues were ultimately seen as private, two questions would remain to be answered: Should it be a public decision whether such issues are public or private? If such issues belong in the private sector, should government adopt a policy or law stipulating as much? If government so acted, it would be adopting the policy that such decisions in our society should be made by private citizens. The *Roe v. Wade* abortion decision was essentially of this type. By striking down the Texas abortion statute, the Supreme Court made the abortion decision, at least during the first two trimesters, a private issue, and was essentially formulating public policy.

Considerable controversy exists over the role of the Supreme Court in formulating public policy. Ronald Dworkin, for example, drew a distinction between arguments of policy and arguments of principle. Whereas arguments of policy justify decisions based upon collective goals or the public good, arguments of principle justify decisions based upon respect for individual or group rights. "A policy [is] that kind of standard that sets out a goal to be reached, generally an improvement in some economic, political, or social feature of the community (though some goals are negative, in that they stipulate that some present feature is to be protected from a diverse change). A principle [is] a standard that is to be observed, not because it will advance or secure an economic, political, or social situation deemed desirable, but because it is a requirement of justice or fairness or some other dimension of morality" (Dworkin, 1977). According to Dworkin, the Supreme Court's role is not to formulate public policy, but rather to justify decisions based upon the recognition of rights. Public policy formulation is a function of the legislature.

David Richards, on the other hand, rejected Dworkin's distinction. "The distinction between principles and social policies seems clearly untenable. Social policies are sensibly regarded as attempts to realize principles of quite complex kinds, for example, principles of justice; and principles of various kinds, for example, principles of efficiency are often regarded as social policies. The distinction between legislative and judicial aims is improperly drawn in terms of the dichotomy of policies versus principles" (Richards, 1977). Whatever the resolution of this controversy, it is clear that simply because certain issues involve individual or collective rights, they do not automatically fall outside the public policy realm. Furthermore, whether the Supreme Court's decisions are or should be justifiable directly by reference to rights or goals, judicial decisions, at the very least, indirectly imply public policies in the broad sense of the term, i.e., government action that affects the public. Therefore, even if the issues in question, i.e., those presented by high-risk research, should be adjudicated by the courts rather than the legislature, public policy on these issues is still being formulated.

One definition of a public policy is a "purposive course of action" developed by governmental bodies and officials "in dealing with a problem or matter of concern" (Anderson, 1975). Several characteristics of public policies should be noted: first, public policies are intended to produce a certain goal, even if not the one explicitly stipulated; second, a policy is a social practice, not a unique or single decision; third, policies are usually developed in order to reconcile conflicting claims; fourth, public policy can be either positive or negative, i.e., it might involve a negative decision by the government to refrain from action in order to bring about some end; fifth, public policies are authoritative in that some sanction or coercion is typically involved.

Various types of public policy have also been identified. Lowi (1964) described three types: regulatory policy, implemented through regulatory commissions that control such things as trade, communication, safety standards, etc.; distributive policies, which allocate goods and services throughout the population; and redistributive policies, which attempt to rearrange or redistribute goods by such means as social and economic rewards. As noted previously, the Privacy Act of 1974 already established a precedent for public policy with regard to personal medical information. The issues of informed consent and level of risk were incorporated into the public domain through the establishment of Institutional Review Boards at each institution conducting research involving human subjects. Further guidelines concerning the use of children in nontherapeutic research were promulgated through the (then) Department of Health, Education and Welfare, following recommendations of a National Commission. There does not seem to be much dispute, at least at the theoretical level, that public policy pronouncements are appropriate to protect rights to self-determination in the medical arena, as well as to protect individuals from harm. It is interesting to note that public policy is here being used to protect individual rights, rather than simply to further a collective goal or provide for the public good. This supports Richards' argument that it is appropriate for legislatures to enact policy based upon principles, and that Dworkin's distinction between policies and principles is a false dichotomy.

How claims asserting the violation of the consent requirement are in fact legally defended, however, is a separate issue. For example, some argue that failure to obtain informed consent is not actually sustained legally unless a harm is also produced. Whereas true violations of consent should be seen as battery, they are in fact viewed as negligence, thereby indicating that one's right to self-determination is not really being protected but, rather, one is being compensated for harm incurred. For an interesting discussion of this point see Katz (1978).

The issues of procreation and child care are more controversial. The right to privacy defended by the Supreme Court in *Griswold v. Connecticut* essentially established a public policy placing such decisions in the hands of private citizens, barring any compelling state interests. Prior to *Griswold*, rights to privacy in specific areas were asserted as part of a broader right to liberty and thereby protected by due process. These specific rights to privacy, however, were simply part of the equation in weighing varying interests. "Privacy as part of liberty . . . had no particular claim to preference and fundamentality, and like other unspecified, undifferentiated aspects of liberty would bow readily to official claims of public good . . ." (Henkin, 1974). With *Griswold*, however, a fundamental right to privacy was established, whose infringement called for "strict scrutiny and could be justified only by a high level of public good" (Henkin, 1974).

It is not within the scope of this paper to examine whether an extended right to privacy is constitutionally valid. What is important for the present purposes is to note that by defending or recognizing a fundamental right to privacy, as opposed to conceptualizing it as part of a general right to liberty, the Supreme Court was establishing a public policy with regard to certain kinds of behavior. More specifically, in *Wade*, Justice Blackmun elaborated more fully on this right of privacy. He argued that "certain decisions extended the right to include activities relating to marriage, *Loving v. Virginia*; procreation, *Skinner v. Oklahoma* (sterilization); contraception, *Eisenstadt v. Baird*; family relationships, *Prince v. Massachusetts*; and child rearing and education, *Pierce v. Society of Sisters, Meyer v. Nebraska*" (Henkin, 1974).

Although future judicial decisions could possibly overturn such a right and open up the range of permissible public policies in these areas, even assuming the existence of such a right, a variety of policies could still be implemented. Without actually proscribing procreation between schizophrenics, requiring sterilization, or restricting child-rearing rights, policies could be developed with the goal of, or at least the effect of, deterring reproduction or encouraging adoption. Similar tactics were attempted by some state legislatures to deter abortion, following the *Roe v. Wade* decision, when it was no longer possible simply to proscribe abortions, except to protect the mother's health. For example, various policies short of prohibition might have the effect, intentional or otherwise, of deterring abortion: requiring spousal or parental consent; prohibiting the advertising of abortion services; requiring consultations or certifications by another physician(s); licensing facilities; requiring performance of abortions only by licensed physicians; requiring measures be taken to save all viable fetuses; requiring pre-abortion counseling of all women, informing them of alternatives; and prohibiting the use of public funds for abortion, except to preserve life or for health reasons.

Analogous policies with respect to schizophrenics might also be devised to achieve a desired goal. Two basic approaches can be identified: policies that would discourage undesired behavior such as reproduction by or marriage between schizophrenics; and policies that would encourage desired behavior such as undergoing screening, accepting counseling, or placing a child up for adoption. The former type of policy acts as a disincentive in that it "raises the costs or lowers the benefits of the non-preferred behavior, whereas the latter type of policy acts as an incentive in that it lowers the costs or raises the benefits of the preferred behavior" (Johnson, 1979). Policies of the first type might include lowering or eliminating provisions for child care, decreasing tax incentives for having children, decreasing free health care for schizophrenic adults and their children, encouraging abortions through a variety of techniques, widely disseminating information about the risks of having children who might become schizophrenic, cutting back on funds for medical health care facilities, or even explicitly permitting the identification of individuals at high risk. Policies of the second type might include providing free screening and counseling services with free transportation and child care, discouraging abortions, increasing funds and facilities for temporary child placement, proscribing public identification of individuals or families at risk, lowering the costs and ease of obtaining contraception, and encouraging adoption by easing state adoption laws, e.g., eliminating residency requirements or a waiting period.

Numerous factors enter into an evaluation of alternative policies, once a desired goal has been decided upon. One is a judgment of which policies will work, i.e., produce the desired behavior. This is basically an empirical question. Another factor is whether a policy of incentives or a policy of disincentives is preferable. Since the latter are inherently coercive, libertarian principles of our society would mandate at least a prima facie presumption in favor of the less coercive policy. Although it is impossible to begin to define coercion here, for interesting philosophical discussions of this concept see Nozick (1963) and Dworkin (1970).

A third important factor in choosing among alternative policies, once the goal has been set, is feasibility of implementation. Who would have to initiate the policy? What form would it take? How would it be implemented? Possible initiators might be the legislature (due either to constituent pressure or a legislator's special interest), the judiciary, the president, or perhaps even interest groups or individual citizens. Before a policy can be formulated about any particular issue, the issue must be seen by some as a public problem for which relief is sought. With regard to mental illness, the problem is usually articulated by others, i.e., those who are not mentally ill. In some instances, of course, this is partly a result of the decreased capacity of those who are ill, but it may often be the result of the stigma associated with being mentally ill and the unwillingness to make this publicly known. Since the beneficiaries of policy alternatives with regard to schizophrenics' procreation and child-rearing rights are primarily the children, the children's cause would undoubtedly have to be taken up by others.

Public policy may take different forms. It may specify particular actions to be performed or proscribed (e.g., screening tests, home visits, financial aid); it may simply stipulate a goal to be achieved by any of a number of different actions, leaving the methods open; or it may merely state who or what authority is to carry out some action. Similarly, it may be implemented as a new law, or as a policy recommendation. It should be noted that a laissez-faire approach is also a public policy, with potential consequences as great as for fully articulated policies.

Conclusion

It has not been within the scope of this paper to discuss specific policy alternatives or, at this stage of the inquiry, to make recommendations. The main purpose has been to elaborate the relatively complex ethical and public policy implications of prospective high-risk research, both in terms of the research itself and the possible information to be gained. In assessing the value of alternative research projects and their methodologies, long-term implications are frequently overlooked. However, some very fundamental questions must always be asked. What public response would be warranted by the discovery of certain information? Would or should our society take action as a result of the information gained? Are certain responses so antithetical to the underlying libertarian assumptions of our society that, even if we knew more, little public action would be taken?

Neither research nor its results can be viewed in isolation from the society that supports it, and it is best if both researchers and society at large consider the implications of research before the issues become acutely pressing. Such consideration becomes even more important when the relevant populations cannot speak for themselves, namely the mentally ill and children. Much more thought is therefore necessary about the ethical and public policy implications of such investigations as prospective high-risk research.

References

Abrams, N. (1979), Child abuse and neglect. In: *Philosophical and Legal Reflections on Parenthood.* Oxford: Oxford University Press.

Anderson, J. E. (1975), *Public Policy-Making,* p. 3. New York: Praeger.

Dworkin, G. (1970), Acting freely. *Nous* 4.

Dworkin, R. (1977), *Taking Rights Seriously.* Cambridge, Mass.: Harvard University Press.

Erlenmeyer-Kimling, L., Cornblatt, B., & Fleiss, J. (1979), High-risk research in schizophrenia. *Psychiatric Annals* 9.

Feinberg, J. (1973). *Social Philosophy.* Englewood Cliffs, New Jersey: Prentice-Hall.

Griswold v. Connecticut (1965), 381 U.S. 479.

Henkin, L. (1974), Privacy and autonomy. *Columbia Law Review* 74.

Heston, L. (1966), Psychiatric disorders in foster home reared children of schizophrenic mothers. *Brit. J. Psychiatry* 112.

Johnson, C. A. & Bond, J. R. (1979), Coercive and non-coercive state policies to deter abortions: A comparative state analysis. Paper delivered at Midwest Political Science Association Meeting.

Jonsson, G. (1967), Delinquent boys, their parents and grandparents. *Acta Psychiat. Scand.* Suppl. 195, Appendix I.

Katz, J. (1978), Informed consent: Legal and ethical aspects. In: *Encyclopedia of Bioethics.* New York: Free Press.

Lowi, T. (1964), American business, public policy, case studies, and political theory. *World Politics,* July.

Macfarlane, J. W., Allen, L. & Honzik, M. P. (1954), *A Developmental Study of the Behavior Problems of Normal Children between 21 Months and 14 Years.* Berkeley: University of California Press.

Nozick, R. (1963), Coercion. In: *Philosophy, Politics and Society,* 4th series, ed. P. Haslett. New York: Barnes and Noble.

Pearson, J. S. & Kley, I. B. (1957), On the application of genetic expectancies as age-specific base rates in the study of human behavior disorders. *Psychol. Bull.* 54.

Richards, D. (1977), *The Moral Criticism of Law.* Encino, Cal.: Dickinson.

Robins, L. N. (1970), Follow-up studies investigating childhood disorders. In: *Psychiatric Epidemiology,* ed. E. H. Hare & J. K. Wing. London: Oxford University Press.

Roe v. Wade (1973), 410 U.S. 113.

Rosenthal, D. (1968), The heredity-environment issue in schizophrenia: Summary of the conference and present status of our knowledge. In: *Transmission of Schizophrenia*, ed. D. Rosenthal & S. Ketz. Oxford, England: Pergamon Press.

Sobel, D. (1961), Children of schizophrenic patients: Preliminary observations on early development. *Am. J. Psychiatry* 118.

Wender, P. H. et al. (1974), Crossfostering. *Arch. Gen. Psychiatry* 30.

Chapter 6

Some Roots, Dilemmas, and Research into Confidentiality

JACOB JAY LINDENTHAL

CLAUDEWELL S. THOMAS

This paper reviews some of the origins and dilemmas involved in the handling of confidentiality in clinical settings, discusses attitudes and values, and considers reasons for the exacerbation of this issue in the modern era. The discussion includes various positions taken by professional organizations in psychiatry, psychology, medicine, and social work, and research being carried out in the Department of Psychiatry and Mental Health Sciences of the New Jersey Medical School.

Psychiatry, as a branch of medicine, is particularly troubled by the problem of "agentry," for whom or on whose behalf does the psychiatrist act as an agent. Psychiatry depends more heavily than other medical branches on the preservation of confidentiality. The many forms of physical problems brought to a physician would not usually lead to stigmatization if revealed to third parties, but the nature of the information transmitted between patient and psychiatrist is potentially more stigmatizing and embarrassing. Psychiatric patients must be absolutely sure that their disclosures will be held in strictest confidence.

Freud (1948) spoke of the formation of a pact between psychoanalyst and patient, noting that "the patient's sick ego promises us the most complete candor . . . we, on the other hand, assure him the strictest discretion . . . this pact constitutes the analytic situation." Menninger (1952), one of the nation's leading psychiatrists, on the other hand, took a more extreme position on protection of confidentiality. He was willing to divulge confidences:

It is true that the physician has loyalty to his patient and a responsibility for treating the professional relationship with respect and honor.

But the doctor also has other responsibilities. He has a responsibility to society, to the hospital, to the rest of the medical profession, and the science. No patient has a right to exploit the confidential relationship offered by the physician *a particeps criminis.* Actually, in a broad sense, the patient's welfare is not furthered when the physician is forced into a position of joining him in concealment of crime. The physician cannot condone moral and legal irresponsibility on the part of the patient and to do so may be actually harmful to the patient.

Frederick C. Redlich tersely summed up the problem: "We psychiatrists want to save the patient, but also we want to save the world" (Powledge, 1977).

Every school of psychiatric thought, in addressing the doctor-patient relationship, places a high value on confidentiality. Psychiatrists are quick to point out that it is not the manifest content of the patient's expression that is of interest, but rather that such expressions are a vehicle by which they aid the patient in gaining keener insight into psychological difficulties. Contrary to many laymen's conceptions, experienced psychiatrists are rarely presented with earth-shattering tales. Nonetheless, both laymen and psychiatrists are becoming increasingly concerned about the extent to which a patient's thoughts and deeds (present, past, and future), once expressed to the physician, must be kept in confidence. However, the problem of confidentiality is not entirely modern; its roots can be traced to ancient medical practice.

Background of the Problem

Thousands of years ago, Hindu physicians who preceded Hippocrates were compelled to follow the precept that "once with his patient he (the physician) must in word and thought attend to nothing but his patient's case and what concerns it. . . . What happens in the house must not be mentioned outside" (Dana, 1926). Hippocrates' Oath subsequently, and to this day, requires that "whatever, in connection with my professional practice or not in connection with it, I see or hear, in the life of men, which ought not be spoken of abroad, I will not divulge, as reckoning that all such should be kept secret. . . ." (Dana, 1926). Lest anyone perceive any changes in the patient-physician relationship, the famous physician L. J. Henderson (1935), wrote in a well-known article: "So the personal relations of the physician with his patients and with their families are still understood, when they are understood, at the empirical level, as they were in the days of Hippocrates."

Such precepts would not have been written had there not always been external tensions from beyond the doctor-patient relationship. Merton (1958) spoke on the problems professionals have in maintaining their professional practices while fending off the community, writing that "every professional association faces the difficult task of trying to reach and to maintain a delicate balance between fulfilling its functions for the community and protecting its professional constituency from exploitation by the community."

Sidel (1961) documented the problematic nature of confidentiality in the minds of the medical community by comparing two views held at different historical times. In 1947, as a consequence of atrocities by the German Nazi medical establishment, the Medical Chambers of the Three Western Zones required every German physician receiving a medical license to take the following oath: "I shall always stand up for the independence of my medical work, and as guidance for my actions shall not recognize any other laws than those of humanity, of love of my fellow man and of unselfish readiness to help . . . I shall not divulge what he confides to me, and I shall keep as a professional secret all that comes to my knowledge with respect to him and his ailment" (AMA, 1947). Ten years later, in 1957, the stand on confidentiality was amended to read: "A physician may not reveal the confidences entrusted to him in the course of medical attendance, or the deficiencies he may observe in the character of patients, unless he is required to do so by law or unless it becomes necessary in order to protect the welfare of the individual or of the community" (AMA, 1957).

Sidel then demonstrated a consistent stringency with respect to confidentiality exemplified by the World Medical Association's Oath of Geneva, first issued in 1948. This Oath, which supplants the Hippocratic Oath in many American and European medical schools, minces no words with respect to confidentiality. It states: "Now being admitted to the profession of Medicine, I solemnly pledge to consecrate my life to the services of humanity. . . . I will hold in confidence all that my patient confides in me. . . ." (AMA, 1951). A year later, the Third General Assembly of the World Medical Association met in London and adopted the International Code of Medical Ethics, which states: "A doctor owes to his patient absolute secrecy on all which has been confided to him or which he knows because of the confidence entrusted to him. . . ." (AMA, 1949). Sidel highlighted the above by quoting a 1954 interpretive statement of the Eighth General Assembly in Rome: "Professional secrecy by its very nature must be absolute. It must be observed in all cases (*"ergo omnes"*). A secret shared is no longer a secret. Exceptions to the rule of professional secrecy can be made only in special cases such as reporting the incidence of epidemic or communicable diseases" (AMA, 1955).

The contemporary practicing clinician must daily make many decisions in the role of agent of either the patient or society. How to resolve this dilemma is insufficiently known empirically. The clinician's behavior may well be determined by the source of financial support. Ruesch (1970), suggested this and added:

As far as loyalties and interest are concerned the practitioner is likely to be more loyal to persons than to institutions because his livelihood is made from rendering service to individuals. The public health-oriented physician is likely to be loyal to the community, state, and federal agencies that support his enterprise, and for him the patient is but an incidental example of a population problem.

Hollender (1960) expressed similar ideas:

Only in private office practice can the psychiatrist be exclusively the agent of the patient. In hospital practice, and especially when the patient has been deprived of his freedom (as in commitment), some of his rights are taken over by others. In these circumstances, the psychiatrist must represent the state, the hospital, or the relatives, as well as the patient.

Ultimately, the psychiatrist is an agent of social control, expected to protect the interests of society by alerting agents of public safety to a potential threat from a patient's behavior.

A Contemporary Dilemma

Despite the abundance of statements on confidentiality, one of the critical lacunae in medical education involves the training of physicians and psychiatrists as to the proper course of action under circumstances potentially threatening to the life and property of the individual and/or society. There are few concrete guidelines for proper professional behavior. Certain notable exceptions do exist, e.g., in orthodox psychoanalysis, which espouses absolute neutrality with respect to moral and legal issues.

The confusion encountered in the training of health care deliverers only mirrors that extant in society at large. There exists the Hippocratic Oath, to which every practicing physician must adhere, which demands that any and all information given to a physician by a patient is sacred and cannot be divulged. Yet, recent court decisions, e.g., *In re Lifschutz* (1970) and *Tarasoff* (1974), indicate that a psychiatrist is culpable for not reporting potentially damaging information to authorities. (As a result, a growing number of clinicians are becoming resentful of the seemingly contradictory demands being made on them from bureaucrats on the one hand and patients on the other.)

How has the present dilemma come about? Even a partial explanation requires an examination of the changing role of the psychiatrist. The mystique of the psychiatrist, once referred to as an alienist, is rapidly disappearing, while more is being expected in terms of role obligations.

The psychiatrist now serves society in ways largely unheard of before the Second World War. For example, as Ruesch (1970) pointed out, the psychiatrist is a member of government advisory groups, has access to the mass media, and, as a member of professional organizations, shapes and reviews qualifications. Increasingly, the psychiatrist is found in court, as well as within the school system, and thus is more and more juxtaposed between the individual and society. At the same time, the increase in related academic and governmental institutions, including academic departments of psychiatry, has further changed the nature of psychiatry. Also, fundamentally influential has been a changing view of the nature of human behavior, which looks more to deterministic causes. The old humanistic guide posts have been untenable for some time, and their efficacy has been lost. This has served to further an already extant anomie within psychiatry.

Ruesch (1970) stated:

In the past, abnormality was judged by comparing behavior with the standards embedded in the humanistic ethics of the 18th and 19th centuries. At that time, norms for behavior were clearly enunciated, tolerance limits outlined, and sanctions for deviations defined. The psychiatrists thus dealt with those aberrations of behavior that did not fall into the province of law enforcement. With the ascendance of the technological civilization and its materialistic ethics, however, the humanistic ideals have become blurred. No longer is the church, the government, the community, or the family concerned with the setting of ethical standards of conduct. Modern institutions have relinquished this task because they erroneously believe that new values will emerge out of technological progress. . . . Today, then, neither the psychiatrists nor the people at large know what behavioral standards should prevail.

While medicine has been received as a humanistic enterprise, civilization has imposed

. . . a split in the medical and psychiatric professions regarding how to implement this humanistic endeavor . . . their personal service orientation. Thus, there are physicians who see service as a personalized business and others who see it as a social and collective responsibility. In the personal service orientation, the rewards for the physician are fees for service; in the public health orientation, the rewards lie in security of employment and inclusion in the group (Ruesch, 1970).

Ruesch also pointed out that the earliest exposure to the demands of society comes during residency training, which takes place in an institutional setting and is frequently funded by a government agency or foundation. Sooner or later young psychiatrists come to the realization that, in addition to being therapists, namely, being charged with taking care of individual patients, they have another role that includes being responsible to the larger society. They are charged with protecting the society from deviants who might potentially disturb the social order.

Brickman (1970) addressed this point:

Psychiatry is never practiced in a social vacuum. Few psychiatrists realize that the charismatic mantle placed on their shoulders has been put there by society, which looks to psychiatrists to perform certain vital social functions related to the control of deviant behavior. Viewed in social perspective, the psychiatrist wears his charisma only because he is an officially recognized agent of social control. He is vested by society with the role of identifying those who are peculiarly disruptive to smooth societal functioning. He is given the power to grant these deviants a social role known as mental illness, thereby allowing them to be exempted from many social obligations. He is then expected to resocialize these deviants in such a way as to return them to undisruptive social functioning. . . . Wearing our charisma, we practice our profession generally as agents of the social system.

The psychiatrist trained today is likely to rotate through, if not receive all training in, a mental health center. Patients seen are likely to be ambulatory and short-term, as well as the recipients of fast-acting, potent, psychoactive drugs. Hence, the humane practitioner who might have developed over time is overwhelmed by the dictates of new strategies of psychiatric care. Importantly, the psychiatrist is increasingly being paid by the system, which is to a large extent informed by the law and prevailing sense of justice. Whereas medicine, at least since the time of Hippocrates, has concerned itself with benefiting the individual, legal institutions have taken the more utilitarian view, namely, the greatest good for the greatest number. In the long run, the resolution of the psychiatrist's dilemma

depends on how deeply modern medical practitioners and policymakers reflect on the profound moral dilemmas and theses of the theory of justice. They must refuse to relax those dilemmas either by a facile appeal to the "inestimable social benefits of medicine," on the one hand, or the "inviolable individual rights of patient or practitioner" on the other. Neither assertion can stand alone; both must be comprehended within an adequate theory of justice. Above all, public policy relative to the shape of institutions, the flow of money and people through them, the regulation of their powers and vigilance over their performance, must be devised with the requirements of justice foremost in mind (Jonsen & Hellegers, 1976).

Consequently, the clinician is forced to engage in an uphill fight to "repersonalize" the individual. As Ruesch (1967) stated:

In a period, in which institutions, organizational enterprises, and technology depersonalize living, the psychotherapist has to fight to put the individual back into the center of political, economical, and biological systems. In order to oppose the trend of molding man in the image of the machine and of creating a world that caters to inanimate things, the modern psychiatrist has shifted his focus from individual to group, from psychopathology to social pathology, and from psychodynamics to social dynamics. Consequently, the methods of intervention have veered from the traditional one-to-one relation to multi-person interaction. More and more does the psychiatrist become an expert in the understanding and management of social processes.

The evolution of biostatistics and epidemiology has changed the concept of medicine within the field from an institution with "limited effects in time and space" to an institution with "knowledge of extensive and perpetuated effects" (Jonsen & Hellegers, 1976). Also, since many costs are absorbed by the general public and insurance companies, what goes on between patient and physician is potentially not as inviolate as it once was.

The dilemma of the psychiatrist is accentuated in some situations, e.g., in the military. On the one hand, the military psychiatrist has usually recently completed training and has the traditional concerns for the patient. On the other hand, the obligation of a military psychiatrist is to maintain or restore the health of as many people as possible so that they can implement the goals of the military. Confidentiality between patient and physician does not exist, and a military psychiatrist who refuses a direct order to make public a patient's record risks a court martial (Clausen & Daniels, 1966). A serviceman may under certain conditions invoke the doctor-patient privilege against a military physician's testimony in a state court where such privilege is recognized. Schwartz (1971) discussed the symptoms he personally manifested as a psychiatrist trying to combine the two approaches in the military:

The author tried to compromise with both by occasionally overlooking certain diagnoses, by underdiagnosing, by overdiagnosing, and assorted wheeling and dealing. Multiple tension headaches, anxieties, feelings of guilt and anger were the results. . . . What possible alternatives are there?

Because of expansion of their role, psychiatrists need not be personally involved in the conflict between the individual and society. Psychiatrists sometimes function as consultants to clergymen, industrialists, diplomats, and educators. Zinberg (1965), focusing on the professional conflicts of psychiatrists in an academic setting, told of one psychiatrist who, once entrenched in the colleges, "found it necessary to ask the college to slow down its demand for his services. Too often a psychiatric referral became a way out when a student presented a knotty problem." For Zinberg, "the professional dilemma of the psychiatric represents the social dilemma of our culture."

The American Psychiatric Association expressed its concern over the issue of confidentiality by accepting a recommendation of a subcommittee of the Association's Committee on Public Information to prepare for psychiatrists a guide for "coping with problems of confidentiality, privilege, and the safeguarding of medical records in their relations with media, business, lawyers, government, schools, and other agencies" (American Psychiatric Association, 1970). The subcommittee's report was approved by the Board of Trustees of the American Psychiatric Association on December 12–13, 1969.

The approved guidelines (American Psychiatric Association, 1970) advised that the primary concern of the psychiatrist be for the welfare of the patient, but included a caveat to the effect that confidential information divulged to the psychiatrist under certain circumstances might be imparted to others. In such an event, divulgence "is to be done in strict accordance with legal requirement and procedures, ethical guidelines, good judgment, and common sense, and always with the welfare of the patient as the underlying consideration." The psychiatrist was explicitly advised never to reveal "except with proper authorization or, if necessary, under legal compulsion—for example, a court order—confidential information disclosed to him by a patient in the treatment process. Consultation with one's own legal counsel may be necessary."

Several years previously, and in contrast, the Council of the American Psychiatric Association had approved a statement of the Association's Committee on Ethics (American Psychiatric Association, 1968) that tended to favor the breaking of confidentiality in the event of a threat to community welfare. Members of that Committee stated:

When in the opinion of the psychiatrist, it becomes necessary, in order to protect the welfare of the patient or the community, to reveal confidential information disclosed by the patient (for example, when he believes that the future behavior of the patient may constitute a risk of future injury to the patient or others), it is desirable where possible to obtain the authorization of the appropriate person such as the next of kin, legal guardian, legal counsel, or by the order of the court. It may be necessary and is ethically correct, for the psychiatrist to take action without such authorization in order to protect the patient and others by preventing the patient from carrying out a criminal act.

Psychologists also have been keenly sensitive to problems of confidentiality. On January 30, 1977 the American Psychological

Association's Council of Representatives approved a document (American Psychological Association, 1977) entitled *Ethical Standards of Psychologists*. Principle 5 discussed confidentiality and suggested that a primary obligation of the psychologist is to safeguard information gained as a function of teaching, practice, or investigations. It stated that "information received in confidence is revealed only after most careful deliberation and when there is clear and imminent danger to an individual or to society, and then only to appropriate professional workers or public authorities."

Social workers have long concerned themselves with confidentiality, at least to the time when Mary E. Richmond wrote that "in the whole range of professional contacts there is no more confidential relationship than that which exists between the social worker and the person or family receiving treatment" (Richmond, 1922). In that same year social workers promulgated a code of ethics, among whose precepts was confidentiality. Currently, social workers consider themselves ethically bound to "respect the privacy of clients and hold in confidence all information obtained in the course of professional service" (NASW, 1980).

When the clinician is forced to choose one course of action over another, what occurs in essence is that "the right of each is pushed into a wrong because it ignores the right of the other" (Sperry, 1948). Such a situation demands ethical action. If, as Little & Strecker (1956) pointed out, the "rights of an individual patient are in opposition to the rights of society, the doctor or the psychiatrist is confronted with the necessity of making a difficult decision which intimately involves his ethical approach to the practice of medicine. In this area, there are considerations about which there is a good deal of uncertainty and divergence of opinion."

The Possibility of Resolution

How can the psychiatrist or other clinician resolve the dilemma? Clearly, the problem involves role-conflict resolution, which refers to the manner in which persons confronted with conflicting prescriptions resolve their dilemmas. There are at least three modes of role-conflict resolution: avoidance, compromise, and preferential selection. Avoidance is a course of action completely inconsistent with all opposing prescriptions; compromise is a course not inconsistent but also not fully consistent with any of them; preferential selection is a course of action consistent with one of the opposing prescriptions.

Reference group theory is one useful approach to the problem. Although most people would probably agree as to what constitutes a reference group, its connotations are described differently. It has been called a group with which one compares oneself when making a self-judgment (Kelley, 1952; Shibutani, 1952); a source of one's values (Kelly, 1952) and perspectives (Hartley, 1951; Newcomb, 1950; Shibutani & Sherif, 1956); and a group whose acceptance one seeks (Shibutani, 1952). Presumably one who wishes to gain and/or maintain membership in a reference group adopts and/or seeks to perpetuate the values of that group.

People frequently have multiple reference groups. A psychiatrist may have the American Medical Association, the American Psychiatric Association, and the New York Institute and Society for Psychoanalysis. In many situations the norms governing these groups converge, giving clear direction to the psychiatrist. However, sometimes the norms do not converge, e.g., when a therapist is confronted with a recidivistic rapist. On the one hand, the therapist is sworn to uphold the Hippocratic Oath, forbidding disclosure of the knowledge to a third party. On the other hand, the therapist is a member of a larger community, perhaps a woman herself, or a man with a wife and/or female children. What alternatives are open?

Stouffer (1949) discussed the dilemma:

If a person has a simultaneous role in two or more groups such that simultaneous conformity to the norms of each of the groups is incompatible, he can take one of only a limited number of actions, for example: (1) he can conform to one set of role expectations and take the consequence of nonconformity to other sets; (2) he can seek a compromise position by which he attempts to conform in part, though not wholly, to one or more sets of role expectations, in the hope that the sanctions applied will be minimal.

He also suggested two important factors: first, adherence to the rules prescribed by the authority depends to no small extent on their compatability with the dominant values of those who must obey them; second, "There may be variability among members of the group in the extent to which a given value is held in common. The existence of such variability is a factor which should weaken the sanctions against any particular act and facilitate compromise solutions." Social research can address this variability.

The following section covers, in broad terms, some of the authors' research into the problem of confidentiality, including past accomplishments, present understandings, and future plans.

Current Research

During the last several years, investigators have begun to empirically examine various aspects of confidentiality in clinical settings. Thus, Swoboda et al. (1978) learned that a high proportion of Nebraska psychiatrists, psychologists, and social workers were ignorant of statutes regarding privileged communication and child-abuse reporting. Jagim et al. (1978) found that a majority of mental health workers, while acknowledging the importance of maintaining confidentiality, were also predisposed under certain circumstances to break it. In addition, while some clinicians favored absolute confidentiality, 95 percent believed that their clients expected communications to remain confidential.

The present authors embarked on a multifaceted examination of confidentiality issues whose results can be divided into four areas. The first area was an investigation of psychiatrists, psychologists, and internists (Lindenthal & Thomas, 1980) and of social workers (Lindenthal, Jordan, et al., 1985). The second area focused on the attitudes of patients and lay nonpatients toward confidentiality as the topic relates to psychiatrists (Lindenthal & Thomas, 1982a), psychologists (Lindenthal & Thomas, 1984), and internists (Lindenthal & Thomas, 1982b), and in light of the rise of the consumer movement (Breslow, 1980; Glogow, 1973; Hatch, 1978; Kunnes, 1970; Melum, 1977; Perr, 1976; Shenkin & Warner, 1973). The third area examined the management of confidentiality in medical school student mental health settings (Lindenthal et al., 1984). The fourth area consisted of studies of confidentiality from a cross-cultural perspeclive, which were carried out in Egypt and Israel (Lindenthal, Thomas, & Ghali, 1985).

Our research involving American clinicians covered all the psychiatrists cited in the New Jersey section of the *Directory of Medical Specialists* (Marquis, 1976), a 50-percent random sample drawn from New Jersey physicians practicing internal medicine, and all the practicing psychologists cited in the New Jersey section of the *Biographical Directory* (American Psychological Association, 1976). The sample of social workers was gathered from a mailing list of the New Jersey branch of the National Association of Social Workers (NASW). NASW members with B.S.W. or Ph.D. degrees were excluded, and a 25-percent random sample was drawn from among the remaining 488 members. Quota sampling was employed to help ensure that samples of lay persons represented the New Jersey population in variables of age, sex, and race. Medical student mental health clinicians were identified through their deans. Clinicians from 59 American medical schools participated. Samples of Egyptian psychiatrists and internists were gathered through the good offices of the Egyptian Ministry of Health, while samples of Israeli psychiatrists, psychologists, and internists were chosen through the cooperation of the major Israeli medical schools and from lists provided by the *Kupat Cholim* or national health insurance system.

A questionnaire was developed for the first area of study with items designed to yield sociodemographic data, as well as information regarding the nature and type of professional practice of the respondent. It also contained ten vignettes, each representing a conflict involving confidentiality that clinicians might confront in their daily practices. Clinicians were asked to check one or more listed categories of potential ways of handling such conflicts and were given an opportunity to suggest additional alternatives. They were also asked to state, in one or two brief sentences, the reasons for their choices. Each reply was independently judged by two raters, who determined whether the response represented a patient orientation, a society orientation, or both patient and society orientations.

The findings revealed significant differences among the professional groups with respect to a stated willingness to break confidentiality. Neither the nature of the clinicians' professional activities nor the proportion of time they spent in various professional settings was related to our dependent variable. This was not the case for clinicians who had had experience with socially threatening behavior. Psychologists who had faced threatening behavior were significantly more reluctant to state a willingness to break confidentiality.

The questionnaire employed in the second area of study was very similar to the one used in the first. Lay respondents were requested to imagine themselves in the place of clinicians and to relate how they as clinicians might handle situations portrayed in the vignettes. Analysis of the data suggests that attitudes toward confidentiality are related to the clinical group to which laymen turn for care and that, in many cases, laymen are more likely than professionals to break confidentiality. In the third area of study, clinicians practicing in medical school settings exhibited a decided reluctance to divulge confidential information.

For the fourth area of study, the questionnaire was translated into both Arabic and Hebrew. Data from the samples of American psychiatrists, psychologists, and internists were included in the overall analysis. The findings showed a similarity in attitude toward confidentiality among respondents of professional orientation, irrespective of country of practice, and important differences across cultures, depending upon the nature of the threat posed by the patient.

When asked to comment on the problems of confidentiality, many respondents cited important concerns, made insightful comments, and offered useful suggestions. One eclectically oriented psychiatrist decried what he perceived as a "double standard for justice":

If I would not have to worry about being sued right and left and if there would not be a "double standard for justice" in our society, I would proceed with direct action whenever necessary without bothering to ask patient's consent. It is regretfully a sad fact, however, that in our present society a physician [i.e., psychiatrist] often is faced with the problem that no matter what he does he might be wrong: 1) If he does not go all out in one direction, he can be called negligent. 2) If he goes all out, he can be accused of invading and/or violating patients' constitutional rights. The "double standard of justice" exists in the form that: 1) If the professional [psychiatrist] is accused of something, he is usually looked upon as being guilty unless he can prove beyond a doubt that this is not the case. 2) If the non-professional and/or the patient perpetrator, etc., etc., is accused of something, he is usually considered and/or looked upon as not guilty unless it can be proved beyond a doubt, that he indeed has a problem and/or is guilty as accused.

Some bemoaned the fact that much confusion surrounds the issue. "Most of us," one wrote, "would not handle the kind of thing you are asking without consulting one or more colleagues and our lawyers." Among the suggested solutions was "a hotline to be called to get immediate advice as to the legality of commitment procedures." Several respondents expressed a desire for pertinent formal training, one writing that "perhaps a seminar dealing with societal and moral issues of psychiatry versus patients' rights should be arranged and soon!" Another echoed these views by writing, "I support efforts to provide a forum to discuss, enlighten, and educate practitioners in collaborative efforts with legal counselors, the court and law enforcement personnel."

Among the limitations of our findings thus far is that they represent only what people say they would do; we cannot necessarily deduce from the data what they actually do (Deutscher, 1973). The data do, however, serve to suggest new hypotheses for empirical research.

Because the needs for confidentiality and disclosure compete with each other, there can be no uniform set of guidelines. Nevertheless, we hope that our research into patient-doctor confidentiality will begin to provide data upon which a more reliable definition of the situation can be established. Giving the parties to the dilemma an opportunity to express themselves may sensitize those in responsible positions—clinicians, educators, lawyers, and legislators—and alert them to options and courses of action of which they may not have been aware. The problem we have discussed also pervades other professions and represents only a specific case of a generic problem of cultural existence.

References

American Medical Association (AMA) (1947), Foreign letters, Bad Nauheim physicians' convention. *J. Am. Med. Assoc.* 135:811–880.

———— (1949). Proceedings of Atlantic City meeting: Minutes of annual session of AMA House of Delegates, Atlantic City, June 6–10. *J. Am. Med. Assoc.*

———— (1951), Hippocratic Oath. *J. Am. Med. Assoc.* 146:793.

———— (1955), *J. Am. Med. Assoc.* 157:245–250.

———— (1957), Proceedings of New York meeting: Abstract of proceedings of AMA House of Delegates, June 3–7. *J. Am. Med. Assoc.* 164:1099–1124.

American Psychiatric Association (1968), Position statement on confidentiality and privilege with special reference to psychiatric patient. *Am. J. Psychiatry* 124:175–176.

———— (1970), Position statement on guidelines for psychiatrists: Problems in confidentiality. *Am. J. Psychiatry* 126:187–193.

American Psychological Association (1976), *Biographical Directory.* Washington, D.C.: American Psychological Association.

———— (1977), Ethical standards for psychologists approved by the Council of Representatives. Washington, D.C.: American Psychological Association.

Breslow, L. (1980), Personal health care. In: Maxcy-Rosenau, *Preventative Medicine and Public Health*, ed. J. M. Last, pp. 1717–1752. New York: Appleton, Century and Crofts.

Brickman, H. R. (1970), Mental health and social change: An ecological perspective. *Am. J. Psychiatry* 127:55–61.

Clausen, R. D. & Daniels, A. K. (1966), Role conflicts and their ideological resolution in military psychiatric practice. *Am. J. Psychiatry* 123: 280–287.

Dana, C. D. (1926), *The Peaks of Medical History.* New York: Paul B. Hoeber.

Deutscher, I. (1973), *What We Say—What We Do.* Glenville, Ill.: Scott-Foresman.

Freud, S. (1948), *An Outline of Psychoanalysis.* New York: Norton.

Glogow, E. (1973), Community participation and sharing in control of public health services. *Hlth. Svc. Rep.* 88:442–448.

Hartley, E. L. (1951), Psychological problems of multiple group membership. In: *Social Psychology at the Crossroads*, ed. J. H. Rohrer & M. Sherif, pp. 371–386. New York: Harper and Row.

Hatch, J. (1978), Self help and consumer participation. *Anns., New York Acad. Sci.* 310:49–56.

Henderson, L. J. (1935), Physician and patient as a social system. *N. Engl. J. Med.* 212:819–823.

Hollender, M. H. (1960), The psychiatrist and the release of patient information. *Am. J. Psychiatry* 116:828–833.

In re Lifschutz (1970), 2 Cal 3d.

Jagim, R. D., Wittman, W. D., & Noll, J. O. (1978), Mental health professionals' attitudes toward confidentiality, privilege, and third-party disclosure. *Prof. Psychol.* 9:458–466.

Jonsen, A. R. & Hellegers, A. E. (1976), Conceptual foundations for an ethics of medical care. In: *Ethics and Health Care Policy*, ed. R. M. Veath & R. Branson, pp. 17–33. Cambridge, Mass.: Ballinger.

Kelley, H. H. (1952), Two functions of reference groups. In: *Readings in*

Social Psychology, revised edition, ed. G. E. Swanson, T. M. Newcomb, & E. L. Hartley, pp. 410–414. New York: Holt.

Kunnes, R. (1970), Community control of community health. *New Physician* 19:28–33.

Lindenthal, J. J., Amaranto, E. A., Jordan, T. J., & Wepman, B. J. (1984), Decisions about confidentiality in medical student mental health settings. *J. Couns. Psychiatry* 31:573–576.

Lindenthal, J. J., Jordan, T., Lentz, J., & Thomas, C. S. (1985), Social workers' management of confidentiality. (Submitted for publication.)

Lindenthal, J. J., Thomas, C. S. (1980), A comparative study of the handling of confidentiality. *J. Nerv. Ment. Dis.* 168:361–369.

_______ (1982a), Psychiatrists and the public address confidentiality. *J. Nerv. Ment. Dis.* 170:319–323.

_______ (1982b), Consumers, clinicians and confidentiality. *Soc. Sci. Med.* 16:333–335.

_______ (1984), Attitudes toward confidentiality. *Admin. Ment. Hlth.* 11:151–159.

Lindenthal, J. J., Thomas, C. S., & Ghali, A. (1985), A cross-cultural study of confidentiality. *Soc. Psychiatry* 20:140–144.

Little, R. B. & Strecker, E. A. (1956), Moot questions in psychiatric ethics. *Am. J. Psychiatry* 113:455–460.

Marquis Who's Who (1975–1976), Directory of medical specialists, 17th ed. Chicago: For the American Board of Medical Specialties.

Melum, M. M. (1977), Balancing information and privacy. *Hosp. Progress* 58:68–69.

Menninger, K. A. (1952), *A Manual for Psychiatric Case Study*. New York: Grune and Stratton.

Merton, R. K. (1958), The functions of the professional association. *Am. J. Nursing* 58:50–54.

National Association of Social Workers. (1980), Code of ethics.

Newcomb, T. M. (1950), Social Psychology. New York: Dryden.

Perr, I. N. (1976), Confidentiality and consent in psychiatric treatment of minors. *J. Legal. Med.* 4:12–16.

Powledge, F. (1977), The therapist as double agent. *Psychol. Today* 11:42–47.

Richmond, M. (1922), *What is Social Case Work: An Introductory Description*, p. 29. New York: Russell Sage Foundation.

Ruesch, J. (1967), Technological civilization and human affairs. *J. Nerv. Ment. Dis.* 145:193–205.

Ruesch, J. (1970). Individual or institution: The dilemma of the psychiatric profession. *J. Nerv. Ment. Dis.* 151:157–168.

Sapir, E. (1932), Cultural anthropology and psychiatry. *J. Abnorm. Soc. Psychol.* 27:229–242.

Schwartz, M. N. (1971), Military psychiatry in noncombat areas: The role conflicts of the psychiatrist. *Comprehens. Psychiatry* 12:520–525.

Shenkin, B. & Warner, D. C. (1973), Giving the patient his medical record: A proposal to improve the system. *N. Engl. J. Med.* 289:688–692.

Shibutani, T. (1952), Reference groups as perspectives. *Am. J. Soc.* 60:562–569.

Shibutani, T. & Sherif, M. (1956), *An Outline of Social Psychology.* New York: Harper and Row.

Sidel, V. W., (1961), Confidential information and the physician. *N. Engl. J. Med.* 264:1133–1137.

Sperry, W. L. (1948), Moral problems in the practice of medicine. *N. Engl. J. Med.* 239:985–990.

Stouffer, S. A. (1949), An analysis of conflicting social norms. *Am. Soc. Rev.* 14:707–717.

Swoboda, J. S., Elwork, A., Sales, B. D., & Levine, D. (1978), Knowledge of and compliance with privileged communication and child-abuse-reporting laws. *Prof. Psychol.* 9:448–457.

Tarasoff v. Regents of the University of California (1974), 118 Cal. Rptr. 129.

Zinberg, N. E. (1965), Psychiatry: A professional dilemma. In: *The Professions in America*, ed. K. S. Lynn, pp. 154–169. Boston: Houghton Mifflin.

Chapter 7

The Ideology of Epidemiological Discourse in Law and Psychiatry: Ethical Implications

LAURENCE TANCREDI

DAVID N. WEISSTUB

. . . Men may construe things after their fashion,
Clean from the purpose of the things themselves.
Shakespeare, Julius Caesar
Act I, Scene III, ll.34–35

Introduction

The past ten or more years have seen increasing emphasis on epidemiological research as a way of obtaining an information base for understanding problems in forensic psychiatry. For example, studies of the determinants of individual competence or threat to self or society seem to have proliferated, and their results are beginning to influence policy and legislative decisions as well as to buttress certain positions and holdings in court cases. A specific illustration is the Ennis & Litwack (1974) article, *Psychiatry and the Presumption of Expertise: Flipping Coins in the Courtroom,* which strongly affected policy and court cases dealing with the role of psychiatrists as experts in civil commitment proceedings. The article reviewed empirical studies of the reliability of psychiatric judgments and conceptual difficulties psychiatrists have in predicting dangerous behavior. The article has found its way into numerous court cases and has been influential in altering policy regarding the role of the psychiatrist in such proceedings.

In recent years, court cases involving forensic psychiatry have increased in number, and, as pointed out by Applebaum (1984), the United States Supreme Court has become substantially engaged with the practice of psychiatry, whereas up until 1975 no Supreme Court decisions had involved "the practice of psychiatry in a civil setting." Since then there have been at least six such decisions. Although psychiatrists and behavioral scientists could once often testify on forensic matters with only limited data to support their opinions, the court and the public now demand more rigor than simple reliance on theoretical constructs such as psychoanalytic principles. One possible response is the use of empirical, particularly epidemiological, studies which, by producing numbers easily packaged into statistical statements, give at least the appearance of being closely aligned with the real world. The intellectual position behind such a response is not incompatible with positivism, for example, which sees empirical science as a means of ordering statements that essentially satisfy such logical criteria as verifiability and meaningfulness (Popper, 1980). On the other hand, one problem with relying on epidemiological (empirical) research may be that data or numbers are often used to avoid the truly hard questions that address broader and perhaps more important conceptual issues. Such a criticism is consistent with the views of Karl Popper; it perceives as a distinguishing characteristic of empirical, epidemiological statements and theories their susceptibility to revision due to critical intellectual evaluation and likely supersession by superior statements and theories (Popper, 1980).

This chapter will explore the broader issues of interpretation of empirical findings, particularly the role of ideologies in epidemiological research, and examine their ethical implications. In assessing the validity of a study, two levels of analysis are possible. First, does the research meet the statistical and epidemiological requirements for a good study? This involves an examination of the study design and methods for gathering and interpreting data. Second, what is the underlying framework: the nature of those conducting the study, dominating ideologies (if any) both explicit and implicit, and the extent to which the research is shaped to reaffirm such ideologies? The discussion will focus on the latter level of analysis. It will seek to demonstrate that the first level of analysis alone is insufficient to establish the meaningfulness of results. The second level of analysis, or critique, is essential to elucidate the influences of ideologies, or preconceived values, on the results of a study and especially on the way data are interpreted.

Essentially, the discussion will treat epidemiological studies in forensic psychiatry as texts with their own metaphors (Lakoff & Johnson, 1980) directed at specific readers aware of basic expressed and unexpressed assumptions—discursive ideologies or concepts, ideas, beliefs, and systematically connected propositions (Romanucci-Ross & Moerman, 1984). This type of critique is particularly relevant to ethics, since the content of information being subjected to ethical analysis is shaped by values that affect the formulating and gathering of epidemiological data and the ways in which the data are applied to the treatment of patients.

Ideologies as Subscript

Ideology is a particularly difficult term to define mainly because it is embedded in a history starting in the eighteenth century that gave it pejorative connotations, which remain a basic characteristic of the concept (Thompson, 1984). However it is possible to define it less substantively, focusing more on how it functions as a neutral process of intellection than on historical usage. To that end, ideology can be considered a body of notions that "transforms fundamental values into action" (Romanucci-Ross & Moerman, 1984). By this definition, ideology becomes an essential condition of knowledge. It is a belief system, not one necessarily fragmented into categories such as political or social, but one that is basic and necessarily inconsistent or incomplete in the sense that it cannot prove or disprove anything about a social or scientific hypothesis. On the other hand, ideologues are able to live with such inconsistencies while at the same time demonstrating distinctions between theirs and other belief systems. Hence in its most ameliorative sense, the clashing of conflicting ideologies (belief systems) may result in higher order ideologies whose explanations of observed events have fewer inconsistencies (Fleck, 1979).

In more contemporary times, ideology has retained a pejorative aura with the writings of Marx, who in works like *The German Ideology* introduced the idea of *"falsches Bewusstein"* (false consciousness) to attack liberal bourgeois ideas. Those espousing Marxist doctrine continue to use "ideology" as an attribute of political and economic positions clearly different from their own and, therefore, subject to ideological corruption. Basic in the nature of this type of ideological critique is the notion of what is incorrect or "falsches Bewusstein."

The Frankfurt School of philosophy has elaborated considerably on the concept of *"falsches Bewusstein"* and constructed its own ideological critique with three primary theses. First is the basic notion that radical criticism of society is inseparable from criticism of its dominant ideologies. Social research then, according to this basic thesis, could have as an ultimate goal the application of critical theory to society. Second, a critique of ideologies must be seen not just as "moralizing criticism" (Geuss, 1981; Habermas, 1968) but as a cognitive process, or method for obtaining knowledge. The critique is not, according to the Frankfurt School, designed primarily to establish morality. Third, such a critique must not follow the epistemological method of the natural sciences but, instead, must focus on disclosing pseudo- or illusory objectivity, make individuals more aware of the origins of their beliefs, and unearth unconscious determinants of behavior. Hence, the analysis strives for self-reflectiveness as a means of going beyond the limitations of objective or empirically derived information to the elucidation of the true interest underlying values and the critical determinants of behaviors and beliefs (Geuss, 1981).

Ideology can also be viewed in a more nonjudgmental sense, one divested of pejorative content. Some involved with the Frankfurt School (Mannheim, 1955) recognized that social thought exists interdependently and coterminously with the political, economic, and anthropological constructs prevailing at a point in history. When viewed from this perspective, ideology becomes a nonvaluative term; any social thought encased in a particular time and space becomes inherently ideological. The objective of an ideological critique then becomes less concerned with evaluating the correctness of a particular position or frame of reference and more with elucidating the values, beliefs, and other underpinnings of the society and social life of a period (Gurvitch, 1971; Edlund & Tancredi, 1985).

Some basic concepts in many legal psychiatric studies lend themselves easily to ideological characterizations, for example, competence, and most particularly, rational consent. How are these to be defined and by what criteria? What constitutes autonomous decision-making and what must be present for that to occur? Similarly, what is meant by notions such as self-determination and criminal responsibility? These questions address highly value-laden theoretical concepts. Examining the term "rational" alone opens up a variety of ideological perspectives. A strong scientific orientation might lead to a strict methodological view of "rational" as meaning the capacity to construct a logical sequence of events leading to a particular outcome. Hence, rational consent would mean that a consenting individual is capable of arranging information in a preconceived logical sequence from which consent naturally follows. However, to others rational might require that decisions be approached in a manner that fits within the norm, that is, the decision-maker behaves in a way consistent with expected majority behavior. The value-laden nature of these theoretical concepts creates almost insurmountable problems for those conducting empirical studies on these questions, that so much of the research must be based on meanings and interpretations of terms pertinent to various belief perspectives.

Empirical research in other areas of medicine often relies primarily on the concrete counting of events and is therefore less broad-based and theoretical than in forensic psychiatry. For example, a study to determine the usefulness of a hospital service from the number of individuals in a community who are using the service would be a well-defined empirical project, simple in design and relatively concrete. Such a research study would present significantly less conceptual difficulty than, for instance, a study of competence in a segment of a medicare population. The latter type of research is more problematic because it has to do with issues of power over and coercion of the individual. That is, the ideology of mental illness, which governs which medical concerns can justifiably override personal preferences or encroach on legal rights, results in studies that deal with broadly based and largely subjectively derived meanings because the ideological framework can be constricted or expanded to slant data (perhaps unknowingly) toward a particular objective compatible with the ideology.

The evaluation of epidemiological studies in forensic psychiatry must consider both external and internal meanings fundamental to the research. In a critique restricted only to external meanings, for example, one might wish to treat empirical studies like a text, perhaps in the sense of a closed text, as discussed by Eco (1984). In such a closed text, the intrinsic interpretation or meaning is so embedded in the ideological base and in the nature of the reader that other interpretations or meanings not only do not enhance the intrinsic meaning but may exist separate from or concurrent with it, or even clash with it. Eco speaks of a text as needing to be understood within the context of a background of codes that may be very different from the one assumed by the author of the work. He goes on to say that, if the author is somewhat indifferent to or does not take into account the different codes particular to different readers, or in fact intends to arouse a precise response from a relatively specific group of readers, then the text is susceptible to a variety of readers' interpretations. Similarly, epidemiological studies or texts can be interpreted in various ways that may ultimately be independent of each other. In "open" texts, on the other hand, the multitude of readers' interpretations are interdependent, and one set of interpretations constructively supplements others (Eco, 1984). Many of the epidemiological studies dealing with highly value-laden or ideologically ambiguous notions are similar to closed texts, and their interpretations depend strongly on the nature of the reader. Furthermore, this variation in textual interpretation with readers' predilections may create major distortions in terms of the scientific validity of the results.

A critique restricted to internal meanings, in contrast, searches for basic expressed concepts and examines the ideological coherence of the framework of the research. Such an "internal" critique includes, at the most concrete level, an examination of the methodology of the research, e.g., the statistical aggregate, the arrangement or cluster of numbers, and the accuracy of mathematical manipulations and interpretations. In the broader sense, an internal critique is concerned with the coherence of the prevailing ideologies from the initiation to the completion of the study. Such a critique is also concerned with the consistency of these ideologies from time to time throughout the course of the research.

Few if any epidemiological studies dealing with broad concepts like competence or autonomy seem to address their ideological foundations. Rarely, if ever, is there an explicit accounting of the beliefs underlying a study, which may in fact vary as information becomes available to alter the operating hypothesis or deconstruct the ideology responsible for the initial design. Despite this lack of explicit identification of underlying ideologies, their nature can usually be estimated by speculation, but closer examination is necessary for greater certainty. Implicit assumptions are usually obfuscated. Once past the first sentence of a statement of purpose, the reader is unlikely to engage in a critical reading of underlying presuppositions.

Most studies begin with a presumption of superiority, that is, implicitly assert the truth of their underlying ideology or belief system; it is their raison d'être. In addition to presumed superiority, some research involves other theoretical beliefs which, although rarely expressed as assumptions, seem nearly self-evident. When sought, however, they are found, and in any one instance may be sufficiently ambiguous or unclear that they fuse with other ideologies and meanings. The first of these unexpressed assumptions is "identity of the framework," that is, the study's consonance or compatibility with some characteristic of truth and reality, especially psychiatric truth as it relates to society (Geuss, 1981). From a pragmatic perspective, one could argue that the assumption of identity of framework is essential for the conduct of any empirical study. If each time research questions arise, one must reexamine the underlying framework of the information system used to structure the questions, empirical research is unlikely ever to be completed. On the other hand, it can reasonably be argued that once the empirical research has been done, the findings and conclusions should be examined against a backdrop of questions regarding the identity of the framework. Rarely if ever is this done in the examination and disclosure of epidemiological research data.

Another category of ideologies, usually unexpressed, is concerned with normative beliefs about the intrinsic aspects of studies. This involves at least four subcategories of issues: first, the framework is the valuable means for empirical gathering of information, that is, the symbols of meaning in mental health —disease, competence, instability, threatening behavior, and autonomy—provide specific examples from the universe of considerations affecting the information to be obtained.

A second subcategory is preconceived notions about what constitutes a good decision by research subjects in any particular instance. For illustration, research by psychiatrists on why patients refuse treatment would probably start with some belief by the psychiatrists of what they would consider a good decision by the patients. Where a patient deviates from that "good" decision, the researchers are likely to request the patient to justify the deviation. Two underlying assumptions apply here: One is that psychiatrists have a clear idea of what justifications would retrieve for the deviant choice the designation of "good decision"; the other is that refusing treatment requires justification. This suggests further that acceptance of treatment would not require special justification, since acceptance is more consistent with the dominant power framework, it would appear "reasonable" and "good" to the investigators.

The third subcategory issue is that research statistics, evaluations, and conclusions are coherent and reasonable. This belief rests on the more primary assumption that the basis for and conduct of the research are truly valuable, and that the framework for interpretation complies with the normative beliefs behind the design of the study.

The fourth subcategory is the assumption of "integrity," that is, the "mind" state of the researcher and the extent to which it is maintained in the text or presentation of the data, the evaluation, and the ultimate conclusions. Some points in the presentation of an empirical study parallel the conducting of it, where internal inconsistencies may reflect ideological incoherence. When this occurs, the "test of integrity" is not met.

Another important broad category of theoretical beliefs about specific research efforts is the "doctrine of error," i.e., an intrinsic concept of what constitutes mistake or false ideology. To be effective, the positive or normative beliefs of an ideology require that error be clearly identifiable. A doctrine of error has its own ideological basis, which may or may not be consistent with the ideology of validity in the research. For example, one study examined denials of mental illness from the perspective of whether the denying patient is truly legally competent to refuse to consent to treatment (Roth et al., 1982). The underlying arguments concerned the precision and accuracy of mental illness diagnoses and of assessments of competence. The authors recognized that denial of illness per se does not necessarily reflect incompetence, that patients may be able to "handle" their everyday affairs adequately and to assess the risks, benefits, and alternatives of the proposed psychiatric treatment reasonably well in all respects but one: they cannot agree that treatment is relevant because they do not agree they are ill. The authors raised the question of whether a patient who denies illness despite signs and symptoms to the contrary should be evaluated as competent or incompetent to decide about proposed treatments.

From the perspective of a doctrine of error in this study, the ideology underlying the diagnosis and labeling of mental illness and the ideology of treatment paradoxically preclude the existence of a doctrine of error. Rather, they create a doctrine of clearly opposing ideologies—that of the treating psychiatrist versus that of the patient who, according to the researchers, may admittedly understand substantive information but deny personal illness. When applying the ideology of psychiatric treatment, one of the two opposing ideologies (the psychiatrists' and the patients') must be dominant. When applying an ideology of what constitutes competence, then the ideology behind the refusal should be closely aligned with the issues of competence. Here it is subtended for the dominant ideology: No ideology or doctrine of error exists to assist the researcher or report reader in the power play of competing ideologies. Denial of illness, despite psychiatrically acknowledged symptoms cannot always reasonably be judged as incompetence. In fact, a test that requires patients to "appreciate the nature of their situation," that is, to accept illness and thereby have no reasonable grounds for refusing treatment, would always assure the success of the dominant ideology. Nonacceptance of treatment would be deemed irrational.

Another study creating a similar dilemma (Appelbaum & Roth, 1981) involved research on fifty newly admitted psychiatric patients to assess their competence to consent to psychiatric hospitalization. Researchers, using several alternative definitions of competence, tested this sample of patients shortly after admission and found that the majority appeared to have severe impairments of competence. The patients were asked fifteen questions on such subjects as their appreciation of the nature of their condition, awareness of the nature of hospitalization, comprehension of the reason admission was recommended, ability to decide to cooperate with the treatment plan, ability to protect themselves in a hospital environment, and awareness of their rights as outlined in materials given at the time of admission. Some examples of the questions demonstrate why a doctrine or ideology of error has been precluded from consideration in this study:

—Do you think that you have psychiatric problems?

—Do you think you need some kind of treatment for your problems?

—Do you think that you need to be in the hospital to get that treatment?

—Why do you think the doctor you saw recommended that you come into the hospital?

—What will the medication do for you while you are in the hospital?

The researchers, in discussing the results, pointed to the fact that half the newly admitted patients did not think they needed to be hospitalized for treatment and that "only 46% could clearly acknowledge that they had psychiatric problems" (Appelbaum & Roth, 1981). This, they concluded, indicated that these patients "were not engaged in the rational manipulation of information that is a desirable element in any definition of competency" (Appelbaum & Roth, 1981). Again, the framework of the questions inevitably led to the conclusions expressed by the researchers. However, the questions themselves precluded an assessment of the error in the research project itself. Consistency existed once the questions were delineated, but the ideological basis for the questions remained relatively hidden though critically important in defining the questions. A negative response to the first three questions and an oppositional response to the last two (attacking the doctor's judgment and denying benefit from the medication cannot automatically be taken as conclusive evidence that the patients could not engage in the "rational manipulation of information," unless one is so ideologically bent as to assume that only one range of responses under these circumstances evidences competence. If such an extreme position is taken, then logically patients would be given only the option to voluntarily accept recommended treatment. If they refuse, they are judged incompetent and their rights can be overridden for psychiatric treatment.

Review of a Specific Epidemiological Study

Of the various epidemiological (empirical) studies of issues like competence, we have selected one to examine closely by an internal critique. We shall abstract certain ideological themes to demonstrate how they are fundamentally integated, not only in defining the purpose of the research but in its very design and implementation. One of the important underlying considerations is the apparent existence of a critical point at which the internal inconsistencies of an epidemiological study (or text, by the Eco analogy) may reflect ideological inflexibility.

The study to be examined is, "Clinical Judgments in the Decision to Commit: Psychiatric Discretion and the Law" (Schwartz et al., 1984). It was conducted in response to some New York State and national court cases and legislative changes that seemed to be grappling with the restructuring or reconceptualizing of ostensibly "objective" criteria for dangerousness to self, dangerousness to others, and ability to care for self. The researchers reviewed decisions to commit or release 90 voluntarily hospitalized patients in a leading academic center in New York State and determined the extent of compliance with the state commitment laws. The study specifically examined the basis of psychiatrists' decisions to seek commitment of voluntarily hospitalized patients, decisions made when voluntarily hospitalized patients filed notice of intent to leave. The study screened every formal request for discharge from July 15, 1982 through November 15, 1982. Individual episodes were considered ended when the patient either eloped, was discharged, was held beyond 72 hours with the filing of commitment papers, or retracted the letter requesting release. Nineteen psychiatric residents were primary therapists for 76 of the patients, three psychology interns for five cases, and three attending psychiatrists for at least eight cases.

The study had two parts. The first requested each therapist to fill out a questionnaire containing 21 items that rated patients from 1 to 7 on legal, clinical, social, and interpersonal variables. The questionnaire also allowed notation of any other factors that influenced the commitment decisions with a rating scale indicating the importance of each factor. The second part of the study consisted of an independent rating of the demographic and clinical characteristics of each patient by the principal investigator.

The results showed that the majority of the patients (66 or 73 percent) retracted their sign-out letters. Twenty-one would have been held for commitment had they not retracted. Of the remainder, eighteen were discharged against medical advice, three were discharged with medical advice, two eloped, and one was actually held for commitment. The researchers compared twelve patient characteristics with decisions to commit or release patients. The characteristics included three legal variables: inability to care for self, dangerousness to self, and dangerousness to others—six clinical characteristics: mentally ill, "in need of further treatment," "understands the need for treatment," "psychotic-not psychotic," "acute-chronic," and "would be a reliable out-patient" —two psychosocial factors: "a place to live" and "support on the outside"—and a single interpersonal characteristic: argumentativeness.

In presenting their results the researchers stated that the study revealed a high correlation between the three legal variables—"dangerousness to self," "dangerousness to others," and "inability to care for self"—and decisions to seek commitment of voluntary patients, and that the legal criteria carried more weight than clinical, psychosocial, or interpersonal factors. They also pointed out that at least one legal factor appeared in every cluster of factors cited by clinicians as having special influence in decisions which they judged as convincing evidence that the legally mandated criteria governing suitability for involuntary commitment were uniformly considered and were among the most important determinants of the decisions. It was concluded, therefore, that the therapists had complied with the law and relied on legal more than medical criteria.

The authors assessed the degree to which clinical criteria might parallel requirements of the law. Here the reasoning became complex and arguably ideology entered into the description and analysis to assure a particular result and interpretation. The researchers saw the legal and clinical criteria as parallel whereas, if anything, they are more accurately described as conflated. In fact they may be interactive and, if not coinciding, perhaps strongly overlapping. The authors' logical error may be that of false cause (*non causa pro causa*), i.e., to mistake the wrong for the real cause of a given effect. More likely, the researchers committed a hysteron proteron, i.e., the logical fallacy of assuming as a premise something that follows from what is to be proved. In this case, clinical criteria are the false cause, and legal criteria are the improperly assumed premise that probably really follows from what is to be proved. The imprecision and potential expansiveness of the description of legal criteria make this fallacy quite possible, i.e., the clinical criteria in the minds and judgments of the decision-makers actually preceded or coincided with the legal justification. The researchers did include a control mechanism, the independent clinical/demographic rating, to check the validity of the clinicians' finding of dangerousness—presence of delusions, paranoia, command hallucinations, anger, belligerence, assaultiveness—but these are clearly medical not legal criteria.

Also, while in the hospital, those patients who were committed required neuroleptics, maximum observation, and seclusion. This would seem to substantiate the authors' argument that legal criteria dominated the decisions to commit. But of course the dialectic could continue ad infinitum as to the ideological basis of the decisions to seclude and medicate. That is, did others not clearly classified as dangerous to self or others receive the same treatment? Or stated another way, the criteria used to prescribe seclusion and medication do not necessarily mean that the recipients of such treatment have met the legal criteria for commitment.

Finally, exactly how the distinctions were made between what is legal and what is medical are unclear. The ideological base biases the distinction. The dominant ideology of the researchers (i.e., that psychiatric justifications for commitment begin with legal criteria) fixes the meaning of the results as a chemical reagent fixes a stain, artificially creating differences where none may exist between what the clinicians conceptualize as "legal" and "clinical" criteria in order to establish a relationship between "legal" criteria and the reasons for commitment of patients. The ideology, therefore, fixes the instant diacritical view and obfuscates the illusory. It enters in to impact on the instantaneity of meaning, even if necessary to distort the results so as to reaffirm the dominating ideology. Hence, it shapes the results in a way that is compatible with affirming the basic ideology.

One could go further, in reviewing this and similar studies, to suggest that the thrust of such research seems always to preserve the underlying basic ideologies. If need be, the objective of the research is adapted to create the illusion of absorbing the ideologies that dominate within the confines of the specific data and study so that the data in fact lead to proof of the hypothesis articulated at the initiation of the epidemiological research. This is an illusion of "difference" created by a specific focus or plane of analysis which, if looked at diachronically, or perhaps from a different viewpoint, would reveal the impact of the ideology on the internal consistency or lack thereof of the epidemiological (empirical) effort. As an illustration of the importance of perspective, a lawyer concerned with civil rights issues, if involved in the same research project using similar data, would be equally justified in perceiving the clinical criteria as including the legal criteria in the minds of the clinicians and, therefore, in arguing that truly legal criteria are not operating as the basis for commitment.

Thus far, this discussion has dealt with some general notions of ideology, especially the way in which particular beliefs function dynamically to create potential distortions in epidemiological studies in forensic psychiatry. We would like now to focus more closely on three broad topics that elaborate the implications of the findings from this analysis of epidemiological research. The three topics are: the role of the reader and the notion of the ideology of error; perceptions of the functions of social research and its implications for this analysis; and the importance of assessing interpretations derived from epidemiological research in forensic psychiatry and examining their ethical implications.

Ideology of Error

Two broad questions underlie a discussion of the relevance of an ideology of error. The first is whether or not it is an ideology. The second is who should be the monitor of this ideology of error. With respect to the first, the argument is strong that an ideology of error exists if there is a system of belief that includes criteria for delineating error. More specifically, in assessing the accuracy of research, the perceiver (researcher or reader) will have an ideology of error to the extent that means are provided to recognize inaccuracy or inconsistency. Karl Popper, the noted historian of science, claimed that a theory is scientific if and only if a full range of observational statements including the "negations of singular existential statements" can be appropriately and logically deduced from them (Kuhn, 1977). When a theory fails in its attempted application, Popper would view this as evidence of falsification. He also stated that the logic behind the accretion of knowledge consists of the investigation of the methods used to systematically evaluate every new idea. From this investigation emerge conventions or methodological rules for the purpose of testing new ideas. One rule, of course, would be that of evaluating the new concept from the perspective of falsification or a doctrine of error.

It may be argued that the application of an ideology of error is simply a mechanical task, akin to applying a doctrine of mistake to any study requiring objectivity where statistically defined parameters exist for measurement, i.e., if inappropriate statistical methods are used, errors will ensue. When the results of a study do not seem to fit into a rational pattern or logical sequence, they may simply suggest mechanical error. On the other hand, when such broadly based philosophical concepts as competence, autonomy, and criminal responsibility are involved, it is necessary to conceptualize sharply what would constitute an error in thinking or in the actual construction of design of the study. The more germane question might be whether a belief system within the text of a study includes the notion of error. It seems that one could conceptualize the doctrine of error as ideological, that is, different groups in a population interested in a specific sort of data might have different notions of error depending on their perceptions of the concepts underlying the studies. Hence, epidemiological studies by psychiatrists for psychiatrists may involve different beliefs regarding errors in research than studies aimed at nonpsychiatrist readers. For example, in a study dealing with denial of treatment and issues of competence, psychiatrists may view error differently than lawyers would. The underlying reasons for the differences in perception may be competing belief systems as much as conceptual error; that is, a mistake, or doctrine of error, would seem to include the possibility of different groups having different perceptions of concepts as they involve any particular set of questions. In social research in particular, which deals with broadly based linguistic concepts, different groups will inevitably have different beliefs about error.

It could be further argued that an ideology of error is essential because it creates the field of interpretation, mapping out the range of "rationally" reasonable and unreasonable results. Hence, if the researcher and the reader differ in their interpretations of the dominant ideology and the doctrine of error, it is nearly impossible to assess the social utility of the results of social science research.

With respect to the second question—who should assure that an ideology of error is taken into account in the assessment of the validity of research—the argument seems compelling that this role is primarily the reader's. Nevertheless, a researcher, such as a psychiatrist doing a project based on a particular ideology, must have an ideology of error to be more than just a polemicist presenting a seemingly rational discourse on a particular position. To offset instinctual stacking of the deck in favor of certain conclusions, an ideology of error with regard to the specific substance of information is essential. On the other hand, a too strongly defined ideology of error may constrain the researcher from engaging creatively in an epidemiological study and taking certain necessary conceptual risks.

From the perspective of assuring the complete understanding of empirical studies, the reader acting as critic stands to benefit most from the application of an ideology of error. The researcher, on the other hand, is forced to anticipate, in both the conduct and final description of the study, who the reader will be. That is, when a study report is presented, the researcher must inevitably direct the results to a specific reader. Moreover, the reader is left with the obligation of defining the underlying meaning systems, present in any piece of research, to be able to perform an ideologically factual analysis. Hence, the reader does more than just gather statistical data presented in a study and attempt to link the data with particular policy positions, but must also identify the underlying perspective or thrust of the study, which requires an ideological critique. In effect, both the researcher and the reader have compelling reasons to understand the scope or spread of their personal doctrines of error. However, since a researcher's sensitivity to an ideology of error might have a constraining effect on a research effort, in the interest of promoting creative work the reader more appropriately should carry the primary burden of examining levels of ideology, including those of error, to establish the validity of the research results.

Nature of Social Research

To some extent, examination of the nature of social research touches on many of the issues already discussed in connection with the relevance of a doctrine of error. The revealing of social reality is probably one of the purposes of much of what is called social research. Some thinkers, perhaps like Popper (1964), would not necessarily take the position that there is likely to be an improving of social reality or of human knowledge. Popper would probably hold that it is not possible to rationally predict the future growth of scientific knowledge. Others, like Kuhn (1970), who posited more directedness in the development of thought or ideas, would probably give considerably more weight to the importance of the process of thought itself in the mechanism of knowing. Categories, relationships, and decisive examples constitute the paradigm that structures the scientist's personal view of reality, of truth (Romanucci-Ross & Moerman, 1984; Elstein, 1978). If the prevailing paradigm of thought on a subject ("disciplining matrix") undergoes alteration, possibly through the emergence of an anomaly that forces a different view, the scientific community suddenly shifts its focus on the affected objects of inquiry as if they are suddenly being seen under a different light. The major change is not due merely to the accretion of new information, though facts continue to be discovered, but is created by the new view, the new perspective. This is significant not only because familiar objects are viewed differently but because interrelationships, categories, and decisive examples are rearranged in a totally new mosaic of data. The accumulation of knowledge has a kind of momentum that is enhanced considerably by paradigm shifts.

Social research may also be examined from a phenomenological perspective, which begins by accepting the intentionality of subjective consciousness understood as irreducible. Phenomenologically, man both creates and is created by intersubjective experience, personal reality (Spiegelberg, 1972). Intentionality is therefore basic to a phenomenological interpretation of what occurs in something like social research (Heller, 1984). From this point of view, social research is concerned not merely with describing and analyzing the reality of social phenomena, but has a proactive role geared toward actually constituting that social reality. If this latter function is granted to social research, it strengthens the argument that a high degree of researcher sensitivity to error and incoherence may disserve the purposes of social research by inhibiting the constitution of social reality in a freely creative way. In a sense, ideologies are stagnant and protective, not expansive and flexible enough to allow creative reshaping of the social reality. Therefore, adherence to existing ideologies could be viewed as counterdevelopment. More diversified types of ideologies might be preferable. If to be effective and good, social research is directed towards constituting reality, then what constitutes reality is simply the limits of our ideological constructs. This would imply that a concern for ideological incoherence or doctrine of error should apply only after the social reality is constituted in accordance with the intention of the researcher. It is this constituted reality that subsequently establishes a guidepost to the limits of ideological incoherence or doctrine of error.

One of the difficult problems with ideological dissonance among different epidemiological studies, or even within studies of the same type, is that once it enters the picture of social consciousness it has a way of altering it. Almost from the moment it appears ideological dissonance alters perceptions and often creates a redefinition of the objects of experience. If an accepted primary function of social research is to reconstitute social reality, then the issue is not so much ideological incoherence or a doctrine of error in relation to the apparent accuracy of the research, but rather a question of a power balance, that is, whether the ideological thrust of the research, in its clash with existing ideological positions, creates such dissidence as to overthrow existing paradigms (Romanucci-Ross & Moerman, 1984). Where social research creatively constitutes social reality, the argument can be made that a doctrine of error has little use except, at the most, to check more egregious types of social research that may reconstitute the social fabric in totally unacceptable ways. This is not to say that a doctrine of error lacks all usefulness in a system where social reseach is expected to reconstitute social reality. However, if limited to the existing paradigm, the doctrine of error may prevent the adoption of any propitious new shift in perspective simply because it is a shift and not because it actually results in a more creative reconstitution of social reality. Some checking mechanism has to be provided both for the researcher in the design of experiments and for the reader in the interpretation and application of the results. Therefore, in accordance with the somewhat teleological Kuhnian model, a doctrine of error is applicable to the extent that it provides, albeit minimally, some control of the reconstituting powers of the supervening ideology. For example, if a research project finds that psychiatrists given sufficient historical information can accurately predict the potential dangerousness of patients, the project cannot totally reconstitute social reality with respect to this particular finding without being subjected to an ideological critique.

This discussion has attempted to address certain theoretical aspects of ideologies and the extent to which ideologies enter directly into the structuring of epidemiological research. Also, ideological considerations were used as a springboard for discussing some notions of epistemology, particularly in regard to theoretical considerations of how knowledge is acquired. The discussion of ideologies, however, was not limited to theoretical questions. It attempted to examine the ways in which ideologies are translated into the practical world of research design, the conduct of studies, and the meaning of the derived information and how it is applied. In this way, the relationship between theory and practice was bridged at least to the degree that an ideological critique could be demonstrated as a method for examining epidemiological research.

Reflection on Interpretation and Its Ethical Importance

An examination of the nature of underlying ideologies and the extent to which they affect the context, arrangement, and interpretation of data is critical at this point in the development of forensic psychiatric science because epidemiological studies are playing an increasing role in informing and shaping policies in this field. Furthermore, ideological critiques are an essential means of understanding when an ideology in this field is false or delusional because of some epistemic property of the constituted beliefs. They are also essential in examining epidemiological studies to reveal unconscious or hidden determinants of the explicitly described research objectives.

Along the same lines, the importance of an ideology of error should be emphasized. A study that does not include an ideology of error in its design is likely to be less an empirical, scientific effort than a polemical exercise. The ideology of error is a type of self-correcting mechanism that is an integral part of any scientific endeavor. Its presence assures some objectivity in the assessment of the validity of scientific results. This ideology is an essential component not only in the mind of the researcher, who must check results to detect and eliminate distortion, but in the mind of the reader, who needs a guide to interpret the results. The anthropologist Devereux (1967) wrote of an anxiety-arousing overlap between subject and observer that impedes the scientific study of man. This overlap is characterized by counter-transference which Devereux said can "masquerade as methodology" and distort the perception and interpretation of data. This observation applies equally to epidemiological studies dealing with forensic psychiatry. Such studies inevitably involve interactions between researchers or "experts in their field" and a patient population. Hence, the potentialities for misperceptions and misinterpretations of data are as powerful as in anthropology and more serious since the results may have major consequences in legislative policy and court decisions. An ideology of error is therefore an essential component of the methodology of the researcher and of the interpretive equipment of the reader.

The ethical implications of the effect an ideological position can have on epidemiological studies in law and psychiatry are especially important because information from such studies frequently finds its way into courtroom deliberations on the rights of patients or criminal offenders. As stated earlier, several important Supreme Court cases involved the practice of psychiatry in both civil and criminal settings. These cases relied heavily on epidemiological information addressing directly such questions as the reliability of psychiatric diagnosis and the ability of psychiatrists and other behavioral scientists to predict dangerousness. *O'Connor v. Donaldson* (1974), the first such civil case in recent years to reach the Supreme Court, relied on information from epidemiological studies that emphasized the tentativeness of psychiatric diagnosis. Barefoot v. Estelle (1983) concerned the ability of psychiatrists to predict future dangerousness; the defendant, convicted of a capital crime, asserted that it was unconstitutional to use psychiatrists at the punishment hearing to predict the defendant's future conduct. In its deliberations, the court considered relevant empirical studies, particularly Monahan (1981). It cited Monahan's claims that psychiatrists accurately predict no more than one out of three cases of potential violent behavior, as well as his conclusion that there may be circumstances in which prediction is "empirically possible and ethically appropriate." Despite their relatively poor record in predicting dangerousness, the court ruled the psychiatrists' testimony admissible, arguing among other things that since similar testimony by lay persons with respect to dangerousness had been accepted, psychiatric testimony would hardly be less accurate.

In *Addington v. Texas* (1979), which concerned the standard of proof required at a commitment hearing to justify confining a mental patient, the Supreme Court explicitly cited the "lack of certainty and fallibility of psychiatric diagnosis and prediction of dangerousness" and concluded that a beyond-a-reasonable-doubt standard is unrealistic for demonstrating that a person is both mentally ill and likely to be dangerous. As in *Barefoot* and *O'Connor*, the Supreme Court relied on epidemiologically derived information to substantiate claims of psychiatric uncertainty and fallibility.

Studies of the uncertainty and fallibility of psychiatric diagnosis and predictions of dangerousness require the same ideological critique applied to the research that indicated that psychiatrists commit patients on the basis of "legally" acceptable standards. Studies of the predictability of dangerousness have not received such a critique largely because they have tended to deal with incarcerated criminals rather than psychiatric patients. Also, these studies have often involved patients institutionalized for relatively long periods and thus acculturated to psychiatric expectations. Both of these factors make it difficult to reach reliable conclusions about the actual ability of psychiatrists to predict dangerousness in psychiatric patients.

Epidemiological studies must be better evaluated because they are apparently used as the basis for many court decisions. Also, the conclusions and recommendations of such studies may be accepted without proper regard for the possibility that the studies may deviate from scientific objectivity because they are influenced by some underlying ideological view. If a study is allowed to stand on its own merits without examination by an ideological critique, certain population groups will inevitably receive unethical treatment by the social system. Distortions, intentional or unintentional, in the design and conduct of a study may escape detection without a well-organized examination for possible ideological bias.

Knowledge can mean power. Those with knowledge of an epidemiological study, especially one predicated on questionable ideological bases, have a distinct advantage over patients or persons enmeshed in the criminal system. Epidemiological information enhances the power of experts in society and creates incentives for exercising beneficent lordliness or paternalism. If the underlying ideology of a study embeds paternalism in its design, and the obtained information escapes critical ideological examination, then a likely consequence is a distortion that tips the power balance in favor of the professional or expert over the consumer. A system of decision-making based on epidemiological studies would maintain the beneficence rule articulated so effectively in the Hippocratic Oath (Veatch, 1981), thereby precluding autonomy in the mental health treatment system.

The ethical issues underlying the use of an ideological critique include the fact that science is rarely neutral. Scientific judgments may be less value-laden than political decisions but still reflect underlying values. If scientific findings are important in influencing policy or other decisions that affect individuals or groups (e.g., patients) in society, the findings create an imbalance and may cause injustice to affected persons. From an ethical viewpoint, an ideological critique can help to achieve a more desirable balance of power between doctors and patients (or police and defendants) by ferreting out underlying, even unconscious, determinants of the overall character of a research project. Hence, the ideological critique tends to enhance patients' autonomy by revealing knowledge about relevant studies and diminishes the exercise of beneficence and paternalism in areas where law and psychiatry come together.

In the study examined in depth above, a logical conclusion of the researcher's results would be that psychiatrists generally abide by legal commitment statutes. By adhering to ostensibly "legally" defined criteria, they are meeting the overall goals of society as translated into legislative enactments. A secondary conclusion would be that mounting concerns over the rights of patients in the mental health system, particularly regarding commitment, are probably not warranted. Furthermore, the study might justify a reduction in the attention paid by the legal and ethical community to psychiatric decision-making in the involuntary commitment of patients. The study also implies that psychiatric discretion in areas of individual rights is probably not as unresponsive to ethical considerations as some have suspected. By extrapolation, even in other areas of patient care, such as the right to refuse psychotropic medications, the psychiatric community may be considered to be obeying the requirements of the law.

However, the ideological critique of this study raises doubts about all these conclusions. It suggests among other things that results are relatively meaningless unless all the elements that go into the construction of a research study are carefully examined, particularly a study that touches on social problems. Awareness of this is particularly important at this point in the development of psychiatry as a medical science. The past ten to fifteen years have witnessed a powerful shift from the psychoanalytical and other verbal therapies of the 1930s through the 1950s to an increasing reliance on biological and procedural technologies (e.g., surgery and drugs). Every year more new technologies are being introduced, many becoming important in the area of forensic psychiatry. For example, chemical castration, now felt to be an important treatment for sexually psychopathic individuals who engage in violent acts, has moved beyond research to recommended use for such offenders in state prison systems (Tancredi & Weisstub, in press). Similarly, the era of psychosurgery (the flourishing of lobotomies between 1945 and 1955 and experimental amygdalectomies to treat violent behavior in the early 1970s—Tancredi & Slaby, 1981) may be upon us again in the near future. The development of more precise stereotactic (positioning) methods, with the aid of imaging technologies such as positron emission tomography (PET) and nuclear magnetic resonance (NMR), is easing some of the concerns about the uncertainty and undesirable side effects of psychosurgery.

Since these new or improved techniques are invasive and aimed specifically at behavior modification, they also offer tremendous opportunities for abuse. Ideological positions regarding acceptable social behavior, individual responsibility, and the relative importance and benefits of psychiatric treatment may considerably influence the design, conduct, and interpretation of studies that might be cited to justify the use of the growing armamentarium of psychiatric treatments, not only to aid patients but to control the behavior of "deviant" persons (Tancredi & Slaby, 1981). The expansion of invasive procedures that alter mood and behavior makes it particularly urgent that studies in forensic psychiatry and other areas of the behavioral sciences be subjected to ideological critiques.

References

Appelbaum, P. (1984), The Supreme Court looks at psychiatry. *Am. J. Psychiatry* 141; 827–35.

Appelbaum, P. S. & Roth, L. H. (1981), Clinical issues in the assessment of competency. *Am. J. Psychiatry* 138: 1462–1467.

Addington v. State of Texas (1979), 99 S. Ct. 1804. (See 1811.)

Barefoot v. Estelle (1983), 103 S. Ct. 3383. (See 3396–3399.)

Devereux, G. (1967), *From Anxiety to Method in the Behavioral Sciences.* Paris and the Hague: École Pratique des Hautes Études et Mouton.

Eco, U. (1984), *The Role of the Reader*, pp. 8ff. Bloomington: Indiana University Press.

Edlund, M. & Tancredi, L. R. (1985) Quality of life: An ideological critique. In: *Perspectives in Biology and Medicine* 28:591–607.

Elstein, A. S. (1978), *Medical Problem Solving: An Analysis of Clinical Reasoning.* Cambridge, Mass.: Harvard University Press.

Ennis, B. J. & Litwack, T. R. (1974), Psychiatry and the presumption of expertise: Flipping coins in the courtroom. *California Law Review* 62, 693–752.

Fleck, L. (1979), *Genesis and Development of a Scientific Fact*, ed. T. J. Trenn & R. K. Merton. Chicago: University of Chicago Press (originally published in 1933).

Geuss, R. (1981), *The Idea of a Critical Theory* (Habermas and the Frankfurt School). Cambridge, England: Cambridge University Press.

Gurvitch, G. (1971), *The Social Frameworks of Knowledge.* New York: Harper and Row.

Habermas, J. (1968), *Knowledge and Human Interest*, pp. 113ff. Boston: Beacon Press.

Heller, T. C. (1984), Structuralism and critique. *Stanford Law Review* 31: 135–140.

Kuhn, T. (1970), *The Structure of Scientific Revolutions*, 2d ed. Chicago: University of Chicago Press.

——— (1977), *The Essential Tension* (Selective Studies in Scientific Tradition and Change). Chicago: University of Chicago Press.

Lakoff, G. & Johnson, M. (1980), *Metaphors We Live By*, pp. 159–194. Chicago: University of Chicago Press.

Mannheim, K. (1955), *Ideology and Utopia.* New York: Harcourt, Brace and World.

Monahan, J. (1981), *Predicting Violent Behavior.* Beverly Hills, Cal.: Sage Publications.

O'Connor v. Donaldson (1974), 422 U.S. 585.

Popper, K. R. (1964), *The Poverty of Historicism*. New York: Harper and Row.

————— (1980), *The Logic of Scientific Discovery*, pp. 49–60. London: Hutchinson.

Romanucci-Ross, L. & Moerman, D. E. (1984), The extraneous factor: Research paradigms in Western medicine. Paper prepared for symposium: Comparing Epistemologies of Medical Systems Cross-culturally and through Time, American Anthropological Association, Annual Meeting, Denver, Colorado.

Roth, L. H., Appelbaum, P., Sallee, R., Reynolds, C. F., & Huber, A. (1982), The dilemma of denial in the assessment of competency to refuse treatment. *Am. J. Psychiatry* 139:910–913.

Schwartz, H. I., Appelbaum, P. S., & Kaplan, R. D. (1984), Clinical judgments in the decision to commit: Psychiatric discretion and the law. *Arch. Gen. Psychiatry* 41: 811–815.

Speigelberg, H. (1972), *Phenomenology in Psychiatry and Psychology: Studies in Phenomenology and Existential Philosophy*. Chicago: Northwestern University Press.

Tancredi, L. R. & Slaby, A. E. (1981), Ethical issues in mental health care. In: *Medical Ethics and the Law* (Implications for Public Policy), ed. M. E. Hiller. Cambridge, Mass.: Ballinger.

Tancredi, L. R. & Weisstub, D. N. Technology assessment: Its role in forensic psychiatry and the case of chemical castration. *Int. J. Law Psychiatry* (in press).

Thompson, J. B. (1984), *Studies in the Theory of Ideology*. Berkeley: University of California Press.

Veatch, R. M. (1981), *A Theory of Medical Ethics*, pp. 296–305. New York: Basic Books.

Chapter 8

The Effect of Law on the Administration of Antipsychotic Medications

ALEXANDER D. BROOKS

One of the most controversial issues in mental health law is the question whether involuntarily hospitalized mental patients should have the right to refuse antipsychotic medications and, if so, what form that right should take. Within the brief span of only a decade the assertion of this quite novel legal right has generated a flood of litigation and provoked an enormous legal and psychiatric literature.

When the legal right to refuse antipsychotic medications first surfaced in the mid-1970s, it was met with alarm and outrage by psychiatrists, especially those who worked in mental hospitals. Antipsychotic medications were, and still are, regarded as critically necessary to the treatment of psychosis, most particularly schizophrenia. All public mental hospitals rely heavily on them for purposes of treatment and control. Most psychiatrists are convinced that giving mental patients the right to refuse antipsychotic medications is an impractical legalism that would seriously impair our capacity to deal effectively with severe mental illness.

Given such a psychiatric perception, why did this critical issue arise when and as it did? How have the courts responded to legal demands? What are the essentials of the problem?

This chapter will attempt to describe the complexity of the legal and medical issues that are involved and to delineate the extraordinary difficulties that arise when judge-made law is invoked in an effort to regulate and exercise control over the medical treatment of mental patients. These patients are surely entitled to some measure of legal protection because the state has exercised its power to hospitalize them against their will and then to treat them with drugs that are harmful as well as beneficial. But what form should legal protection take? Because of the enormous scope of the problem, the discussion here will focus particularly on two major cases, *Rogers v. Commissioner* (1983) in Massachusetts and *Rennie v. Klein* (1979) in New Jersey.

Background of the Problem

To put this legal controversy in context it is necessary to begin with a consideration of the antipsychotic medications themselves, their benefits, and their harms.

These powerful medications came to light only in the early 1950s, when drugs being tested for other purposes were unexpectedly found to have antipsychotic effects. A period of great euphoria ensued among psychiatrists when they realized that with these medications many formerly untreatable schizophrenic patients could be "restored" from their delusions, hallucinations, and agitation toward more normal perception and behavior. As a result of the benefits of these medications, many patients were released from hospitals into the community. Other patients, who were compelled to remain in the hospital, tended to function on a more rational level. The atmosphere in mental hospitals was transformed. The violence and disruption previously created by agitated patients was sharply curtailed. Staff became less brutal as patients was sharply curtailed. Staff became less brutal as patients became less assaultive, and patients benefited from a more beneficent atmosphere.

Mental hospital populations began to drop markedly, as deinstitutionalization, facilitated by the medications, progressed, and have remained relatively low ever since. In one decade alone, the population of hospitalized mental patients fell by over 75 percent (*Western New England Law Review*, 1984). Moreover, periods of hospitalization became shorter because medications tend to attack acute mental problems more rapidly than do other forms of psychiatric treatment. As recently as 1971, for example, a typical hospital stay was 44 days; by 1975 it was only 26 days (Klerman, 1979) and is now even shorter.

Small wonder, then, that psychiatrists, especially those working in mental hospitals, began to depend heavily, often exclusively, on the use of antipsychotics. Many of them still think that medications are virtually a panacea, the "be all and end all" of hospital management.

It took years before psychiatrists acknowledged the limitations of antipsychotic medications. Many patients relapsed, levels of social functioning remained low, and most were not really restored to health but became more manageable. But hospital staff were grateful for the manageability of previously difficult patients.

More seriously, it was discovered that all antipsychotic medications can have strong adverse side effects. Little attention was paid to these side effects at first, although they began to surface soon after the medications went into large-scale use. Gradually, however, an awareness developed among the more sensitive and thoughtful psychiatrists that antipsychotic medication side effects are significant in a substantial proportion of cases.

These side effects are physical, emotional, cognitive, and social (Halleck, 1978). The spectrum of physical side effects ranges literally from dry mouth to death. One of the most common is a condition known as akathisia, marked by an irresistible physical restlessness that often causes the patient to pace interminably and makes arms, legs, and feet shake. Akathisia is also manifested by panic or intense anxiety. Unfortunately, inexperienced or incompetent doctors have often misconstrued such medication-caused behavior as evidence of a continuing psychotic condition and administered even more medication, thereby aggravating rather than relieving the patient's agitation.

Another side effect, with entirely different consequences, is akinesia, characterized by extreme drowsiness. Patients who suffer from this condition report that they feel like zombies, lifeless, with severely diminished spontaneity and extreme fatigue. Many feel they are "sleeping their lives away." Listlessness and apathy make their lives seem empty and aimless, hardly worth living.

Side effects also include such physical problems as blurring of vision, low blood pressure, constipation, skin rashes, palpitations, faintness, and an inability of men to ejaculate. Patients get the shakes and develop blank facial expressions or uncontrollable grimaces, stiffness of gait, leg jiggling, and eye rolling.

Cognitive side effects include an inability to read, concentrate, or even speak clearly. Mental patients may withdraw into an intellectual vacuum.

Moreover, adverse social consequences flow from these conditions. Patients who are sad, morose, and hopeless find it difficult to enjoy adequate social relationships even with fellow patients, let alone with "normals" in the community. Difficulties in social interaction tend to further withdrawal, isolation, depression, and despair.

These side effects, however, grave as they are for many mentally ill persons, pale in significance compared to the most serious side effect of all, tardive dyskinesia. This is a disablement characterized by bizarre and uncontrollable movements of the face, tongue, mouth, and limbs, which are enormously humiliating to afflicted patients. An even more distressing aspect is that it is irreversible for many long-term medication users and is discovered only when it has already become severely disabling. Unlike other side effects, which disappear when medication is discontinued, tardive dyskinesia remains. It has no known cure, although some cases of apparent spontaneous remission have been reported.

Tardive dyskinesia tends to affect long-term users of medications more than short-term users. Among long-term users the incidence seems to be high, reportedly ranging from 25 to 50 percent (Brooks, 1980). As yet, however, little is known about tardive dyskinesia, and much is controversial, including its incidence, its controllability, when it appears, and who is likely to get it.

Patients respond to medications in a variety of ways. Most tolerate them because they realize there is no alternative if they are to be free of mental illness, but they pay a high price in adverse effects on their quality of life. For this reason, some patients find the side effects intolerable. They resist medication when they can, risking decompensation, rehospitalization, and even physical violence—their own as well as retaliatory violence. But most refusers ultimately reaccept their medications, and many repeat cycles of refusal and acceptance.

Psychiatrists typically belittle the significance of side effects by pointing out that some can be alleviated by countermedications and most, but not all, are temporary in that they vanish if medication is discontinued. But chronic patients on a maintenance program cannot discontinue their medications. Their distressing side effects are, for all practical purposes, a permanent condition.

In sum, antipsychotic medication side effects are serious. They are more distressing for some patients than for others, but create a high order of distress for many users. There may be controversy about the nature, extent, and scope of side effects, or such aspects as whether some forms of tardive dyskinesia are irreversible, but the fact remains, as the Third Circuit Court of Appeals has said, "Such injuries occur often enough to be of deep concern" (*Rennie v. Klein*, 1981). That basic fact is not likely to change as long as the current class of antipsychotic drugs is used to control psychotic conditions.

What do hospital staff do to minimize side effects or maximize benefits? The unavoidable biological damage is a grave problem even when the antipsychotic medications are competently and sensitively administered, and careful attention is paid to the needs of each patient. The psychiatric conditions affected by these powerful chemicals are complex, mysterious, and highly individualized. Each mentally ill person responds differently to different chemicals and dosages. Many trials are sometimes necessary before a medication regimen is properly stabilized. Effective and successful administration requires that the attending doctors have knowledge, skill, and patience. But these are qualities in short supply in public mental hospitals where doctors tend to be ill-trained, unskilled and notably lacking in the patience and solicitude necessary for the most judicious use of potent medications.

When antipsychotic medications are administered incompetently, callously, or even abusively, their curative power is diminished and their side effects unnecessarily aggravated. Yet recent litigation and legislative investigations reveal that the administration of antipsychotic medications in public mental hospitals is strikingly substandard (Gelman, 1983–1984). It is not uncommon for medications to be given to patients who don't need them, thus creating the risk of side effects without any possible benefit. This occurs when a patient is incorrectly diagnosed as schizophrenic. Avoidable injury is inflicted also when medications are administered only to sedate or agitated patients, when other, less harmful forms of treatment might be as effective and preferable for the patients' well-being. Too much or too many different medications are often used, a practice known as polypharmacy, which multiplies side effects without increasing benefits.

In some hospitals, medications are used to punish rather than treat patients. When patients complain, the unnecessary medications are sometimes deliberately increased. For example, in one reported instance, when a patient complained about a specific drug with particularly unpleasant side effects, instead of experimenting with a different drug the doctor doubled the dosage (Gelman, 1983–1984).

Hospital records containing critical information about dosage and side effects are often lost. Doctors tend to ignore side effects and frequently claim that patients exaggerate or even invent them. What is particularly remarkable is the extent to which, during the twenty-five-year period from the mid-1950s to the late 1970s, hospital psychiatrists either entirely denied the existence of significant side effects or denigrated both the harm caused by the medications and the reasonableness of patient resistance to them. Even the few psychiatrists who acknowledged the side effects tended to deny the need to take them into consideration, emphasizing the benefits and playing down the physical, emotional, and mental costs. On the other hand, lawyers who later became involved tended to emphasize the adverse side effects and belittle the benefits of medications, much to the annoyance of doctors.

Denial of side effects was particularly common in connection with tardive dyskinesia. For example, when the medical director of a major New Jersey state hospital was first asked about the extent of tardive dyskinesia at his hospital, he claimed that none of his patients suffered from it. Later, when placed under oath in *Rennie v. Klein*, he estimated an incidence of 25–40 percent (Gelman, 1983–1984).

In several litigations, judges reluctantly concluded that state mental hospitals administered medications in a "grossly irresponsible" manner, often for the convenience of the staff or for punishment rather than for legitimate treatment (*Rennie v. Klein*, 1979).

Lawyers Enter the Picture

Lawyers representing mental patients on other legal issues became aware of antipsychotic drug problems in the early 1970s when their mental patient clients complained to them about the adverse effects of the medications they were compelled to take. The lawyers at first pooh-poohed the complaints, crediting the received wisdom that the medications were entirely beneficial, but soon realized that they were confronted with a legal and psychiatric hornet's next.

In 1975 and 1977, litigations were undertaken in federal courts in Massachusetts and New Jersey, respectively, challenging compulsory medication. The lawyers chose the federal courts as a forum because they had decided to assert an entirely new right to refuse medications on the basis of the federal constitutional right to "privacy." Essentially they invoked the right of autonomy, the right of an individual, even though mentally ill and involuntarily hospitalized, to make decisions about medical treatment, especially when potentially harmful. The constitional right to privacy was first established in the celebrated abortion case in which the United States Supreme Court ruled that a pregnant woman has an absolute right to abort her fetus within the first trimester of pregnancy. In general, this recognized the right of self-determination about what could be done to one's body. Patients' lawyers reasoned that a mentally ill person, in spite of being confined to a mental hospital, should have the right to refuse harmful medications even if a benefit was intended.

Three or more major institutional rights were theoretically available to support the patients' cases, each addressing the problem in a different way. However, only one was actually asserted—a federal constitutional right of patients to prevent doctors, acting on behalf of the state, from imposing medications against the patients' will. An alternative remedy, not chosen at the time, was the constitutional right to quality of care in the administration of medications. This would have taken the form of a "right to treatment," of a quality regarded as acceptable by the leaders of the psychiatric profession. However, this would not have included a right to refuse treatment; it presumed acceptance but insisted on suitable quality. Another alternative was the right to protection from harm, already recognized by the United States Supreme Court in other contexts. As it turned out, it was the right to refuse that held the imagination of lawyers at the outset and prevailed for years.

The assertion of a constitutional right to refuse had two objectives. The first was to guarantee patient autonomy, the principle that a patient competent to make rational choices, even though mentally ill and involuntarily hospitalized, has the right to decide whether or not to accept potentially harmful medications.

Such autonomy would include the right to refuse even "perfectly" administered medication, correctly selected and given in precisely adjusted dosages, with all reasonable precautions taken to eliminate or mitigate side effects. As the patient's lawyer in the *Rogers* case put it, "The focus . . . was the right of patients to decide for themselves whether the risks outweigh the benefits of drug treatment" (Doudera & Swazey, 1982, p. 60).

Some patients' lawyers had a second objective, the maximization of quality of care. The lawyers were well aware that the level of medication administration in many state hospitals was extremely poor. In many instances, a patient's refusal of a drug indicated not a general unwillingness to accept medication but a resistance to taking a particular offensive drug or harmful dosage, or a protest at the lack of precautions taken to avoid side effects.

For example, in a New Jersey patient refusal case that immediately preceded *Rennie*, ensuing litigation denied the patient's right to refuse. After the litigation was over, it was revealed that the patient had not intended to refuse any and all medications, only one that was particularly obnoxious. The patient later accepted another drug without further resistance (In re B, 1977).

Was the choice of right and remedy significant? It is arguable that if, at the outset of the *Rennie* and *Rogers* litigations, the patients' lawyers had asked for a right to quality of care rather than a right to refuse, the lawsuits might not have provoked such an adverse reaction from the psychiatric profession. Many psychiatric leaders acknowledged the poor quality of care in public mental hospitals and urged improvement by legal means if necessary, but felt that their most successful mode of treatment was seriously threatened by the right to refuse. Their counterattack was bitter, and ultimately successful in the United States Supreme Court.

Both *Rogers* and *Rennie* involved lengthy trials in which numerous witnesses and documents were presented. The trial judges seemed appalled by the unexpected evidence of the risks involved in the use of antipsychotic drugs and of the incompetent and abusive way in which the drugs were administered. In both cases the judges declared that there was indeed a federal constitutional right to refuse antipsychotic medications. The two judges' decisions were similar as to legal theory but applied markedly different remedies.

Both acknowledged that a right to refuse treatment should have reasonable limitations and could be overridden in three situations: where the refusing patient was dangerous to self or others while in the hospital; where the patient was mentally incapable of making a rational treatment decision; and in an emergency. Otherwise, said both judges, the patient should literally have the power to prevent the hospital from administering medications.

The lawyers and judges in both cases recognized that if limitations or exceptions to the constitutional right were too broadly defined, exceptions could swallow up the right. Patients' lawyers argued for strict and limited definitions of such terms as "dangerousness," "incapacity," and "emergency." Lawyers for the state, on the other hand, insisted that definitions which were too limited would deny mental health professionals the flexibility they needed in treating highly volatile or violent patients. In *Rogers*, for example, state lawyers argued that an emergency justifying compulsory medication should include active deterioration of a patient's mental condition when medication might prevent deterioration. Patients' lawyers fought this proposed definition, arguing that such an exception would give doctors too much latitude and be too easily abused. The patients' lawyers won that skirmish in court. An emergency was defined strictly as a likelihood that an unmedicated patient would engage in physical violence.

Both judges also ruled that the least restrictive or intrusive alternative test should apply, that is, a mental health professional preparing to administer a particularly intrusive form of treatment must first consider whether a less intrusive form of treatment would not be equally or sufficiently efficacious and less threatening or harmful to a patient's liberty interests. For example, an agitated patient might prefer several hours in seclusion to calm down rather than a long-lasting drug like prolixin decanoate whose distressing side effects last for several weeks. One of the major values of the least intrusive alternative is that it tends to prevent mental health professionals from making easy, routine, and automatic decisions without sufficient consideration of their impact on the patient. Thus, even in a genuine emergency, the administration of medication would be subject to a least intrusive alternative test.

Even more controversial were the procedures chosen by the

courts to insure that the right would be effectively respected and not disregarded in practice. The New Jersey judge rejected as inadequate regulations hastily devised and adopted by the state, ruling instead that, in cases of patient refusal, the hospital should hold an informal hearing presided over by a so-called independent psychiatrist who had no formal connection with the state. In addition, each refusing patient would be represented by an advocate who did not have to be a lawyer. The independent psychiatrist, after considering the factors outlined by the court, would decide whether or not the patient's refusal should be honored and was authorized to affirm or reject the refusal, or to recommend a modification of treatment.

The Massachusetts procedures were more formidable and formalistic, requiring that the competence or incompetence of a refusing patient be determined by a judge who would decide for an incompetent patient whether to accept medications or not. A patient judged incompetent would have a right to a legal guardian.

The *Rennie* and *Rogers* decisions generated consternation in the psychiatric community, especially in Boston where leading psychiatrists associated with prestigious mental hospitals and medical schools immediately launched an attack on the newly announced right as unrealistic, impractical, and counterproductive (Appelbaum & Gutheil, 1979). Both decisions were appealed. In the meantime, lawyers in other jurisdictions, impressed with the success of the New Jersey and Massachusetts cases, undertook similar law suits, most of which were equally successful in establishing the right to refuse.

On appeal, the First and Third Federal Circuit Courts affirmed a constitutional right to refuse but significantly modified the earlier *Rennie* and *Rogers* rulings. First, the Third Circuit Court changed the constitutional basis for the right of refusal from privacy, or autonomy, to the right to freedom from unjustified intrusions on personal security. Second, it rejected the trial judge's standards and procedures and reinstated the state's pre-existing regulations, which the judge had rejected. These regulations authorized the hospital director to override the patient's constitutional right to refuse in four situations. The first was an emergency, when medication is necessary to prevent either death or other "serious consequences," not further defined. The second was where the patient is "incapable, without medication, of participating in any treatment plan available at the hospital that will give him a realistic opportunity of improving his condition." The third was where an unmedicated patient would be dangerous either to self or to others. The fourth was where medications "would probably improve the patient's condition within a significantly shorter time" than alternative treatments.

In addition to these substantive bases for overriding a refusal, the legally approved New Jersey Administrative Bulletin provided for procedural stages through which a refusal would travel, which included, first, a meeting with the treating doctor who attempts to explain to the patient why the medication should be accepted and describes benefits and risks. If the patient continues to refuse, the refusal next goes before a treatment team, which attempts to formulate a treatment plan acceptable to the patient. If the patient still refuses, and is legally incompetent, an effort is made to obtain consent from the guardian. If the guardian refuses, the Chief Executive Officer of the hospital is authorized to order the administration of medication after the Medical Director or a designee has conducted an examination of the patient, reviewed the record, and agreed with the treating physician.

If, however, the patient is legally competent, the Executive Director of the hospital can still order the medicine to be administered if one of the four situations described above exists: emergency; dangerousness; incapacity; or comparatively slow improvement. The Third Circuit also affirmed the district court's ruling that treatment personnel should be guided by the least intrusive alternative principle.

The First Circuit Court also affirmed a constitutional right to refuse treatment in *Rogers* but significantly modified the decision of the district court. The district court had narrowly defined emergency; the Circuit Court broadened the definition. The district court, accepting the plaintiff's approach, had defined an emergency as "circumstances in which a failure to [forcibly medicate] would bring about a substantial likelihood of physical harm to the patient or others." The state had insisted that such a definition was "overly rigid and unworkable." The Circuit Court now agreed that the term emergency should also include situations where the immediate administration of drugs is believed necessary to prevent further deterioration of the patient's mental health. Said the Circuit Court, "It cannot be said that the interests of the patient himself would be furthered by requiring responsible physicians to stand by and watch him slip into possibly chronic illness while awaiting an adjudication of incompetency." In vacating the district court's definition of emergency, the Circuit Court urged the district court to consider "alternative means for making legal incompetency determinations in situations where any delay could result in significant deterioration of the patient's mental health."

The First Circuit Court also set aside as "simplistic" the district court's definition of dangerousness, which the higher court characterized as requiring a showing of a quantitative likelihood that violence would occur if medications were not administered. The Court ruled that a medication decision designed to avoid violence should result from a determination that in a particular situation the need to prevent violence outweighs the possibility of harm to the medicated individual.

The Circuit Court also clarified a district court ruling that had been interpreted as requiring the legal guardian of an incompetent patient to make drug decisions for the patient. Said the Court, "The state is not required to seek individualized guardian approval for decisions to treat incompetent patients with antipsychotic drugs." The Court held that hospital doctors should be authorized to medicate a refusing but judicially incompetent patient if a "substituted consent" approach were used. In other words, the treating doctor should attempt to make a treatment decision for the patient as the patient himself or herself would make it if competent. The Court suggested procedures to implement this approach, such as periodic review by nontreating physicians.

The Circuit Court decisions in *Rogers* and *Rennie* were announced late in 1980 and in mid-1981. In June 1982 both decisions were appealed to the U.S. Supreme Court just as it was deciding another case, *Youngberg v. Romeo* (1982), which, though dealing with a separate issue, was to have a great impact on the constitutional right to refuse.

Youngberg v. Romeo concerned a profoundly retarded resident of Pennhurst, an institution for the retarded, who was injured and also shackled by staff to curb his assaultive behavior. Romeo petitioned for a constitutionally protected right to safety, to freedom from unreasonable restraint, and to training. The Supreme Court acknowledged the first two rights and also the third right to the extent that training would be aimed at ensuring Romeo's physical safety and capacity to enjoy freedom from restraint.

In the course of affirming these rights, the Supreme Court addressed itself to the test by which state compliance with constitutional standards should be measured. It indicated that the interest of retarded persons in freedom from restraint and danger should be balanced against the legitimate interests of the state, which include a right to operate institutions for the retarded without excessive burdens, without "interference" from federal courts, and without hospital professionals being forced to make treatment decisions "in the shadow of an action for damages." The Supreme Court wanted to ensure that the legal implementation of a constitutional right would not "restrict unnecessarily the exercise of professional judgment as to the needs of residents."

The Supreme Court held that in court reviews of the validity of doctors' decisions, the constitution requires only a finding that the doctors in fact exercised "professional judgment." It follows, said the Court, that it is not appropriate for courts to specify which of several professionally acceptable choices should have been made by doctors in treating or managing the mentally retarded in institutions. Said the Supreme Court, "We emphasize that courts must show deference to the judgment exercised by a qualified professional." Finally, a "decision, if made by a professional, is presumptively valid; liability may be imposed only when the decision by the professional is such a substantial departure from accepted professional judgment, practice or standards as to demonstrate that the person responsible actually did not base the decision on such a judgment."

Later, the Supreme Court, in reviewing *Rennie* and *Rogers* refused to decide whether patients have a constitutional right to refuse medications. It vacated the decisions by both the First and Third Circuits. It remanded *Rennie* to be reconsidered by the Third Circuit in light of *Romeo* and directed that the Massachusetts Supreme Court be given an opportunity to decide the issues in *Rogers*.

The Third Circuit on remand regarded the Supreme Court's *Romeo* decision as requiring only one significant change in its previous *Rennie* decision. A new majority of the Third Circuit viewed the Supreme Court's language in *Romeo* as a tacit disapproval of the least restrictive alternative approach, which they had previously adopted. They then eliminated the least restrictive alternative test from the factors to be considered in evaluating patient refusals. Otherwise, their decision in the *Rennie* case remained intact.

But the language of the Supreme Court had not been crystal clear. It had not specifically mentioned the least restrictive alternative test, nor were any least restrictive alternative cases cited. The Supreme Court's alleged repudiation of the test was purely inference, although—in context—a strong one. In the event, four of the nine Third Circuit judges were not convinced and held fast to their original support of the test; one expressed the review that a professional judgment that did not take a least restrictive alternative into account was not truly a professional judgment.

As of this writing, several post-*Romeo* federal right-to-refuse cases have been decided. In *Project Release v. Prevost* (1983), the prestigious Second Circuit Court of Appeals ruled that the so-called constitutional right to refuse requires only that a professional judgment be made as to the need to compel medication in order to override a refusal and that New York State's three levels of procedural review satisfy constitutional requirements of due process. In *R.A.J. v. Miller* (1984), a federal district court rejected a mental patient's right to more than a review of a refusal. Finally, in *Stensvad v. Reivitz* (1985), a Wisconsin federal district court, upholding Wisconsin's rejection of a right to refuse, quoted *Romeo* in stating that a patient's "constitutional right to refuse antipsychotic drugs must be measured by whether the decision to administer such drugs is a substantial departure from accepted professional judgment, practice, or standards."

It now appears that the constitutional right to refuse medications has been severely trimmed and transformed following the Supreme Court's decision in *Romeo*. The right has become a right to protest or object and to have an original treatment decision reviewed. Although referred to as such, it seems no longer to be a right to refuse, if by refusal is meant the power to prevent the state from forcibly medicating a patient except within reasonably well-defined exceptions for dangerousness and incapacity.

How has the right to refuse worked in practice? Evidence gathered in New Jersey suggests that it has significantly eroded. The number of refusal hearings has steadily declined since the *Rennie* decision. It is alleged that coercive acts, including threats, are again being used in hospitals to compel patients to accept medications, but these allegations have not been substantiated. In at least one hospital, the Patient Advocate offers no assistance to refusing patients until they have persisted through all procedural stages up to the Medical Director. Most patients succumb to medication pressure long before they ever meet the Patient Advocate (N.J. Public Advocate, 1982, 1983).

On the other hand it is claimed, though with little supporting data, that, although the right to refuse is now only a paper right in New Jersey, the publicity surrounding right-to-refuse litigation and the efforts of the State to regulate its mental hospitals have resulted in a much higher quality of care. If so, the *Rennie* case has achieved a meaningful success even if not in the form of a right to refuse intended by its progenitor.

In Massachusetts, and perhaps in other states, the right to refuse seems to be flourishing as a legal doctrine. Whether it flourishes in practice remains to be studied. Eighteen months after the Supreme Court remanded *Rogers*, the Massachusetts Supreme Court decided *Rogers v. Commissioner* (1983), which turned out to be highly protective of patients' rights. The Massachusetts Supreme Court ruled that, except for emergencies involving prospective dangerousness, a mental patient has a right to refuse medications unless incompetent to make a treatment decision, and incompetence is to be decided only by a court, not by hospital personnel. The Massachusetts court suggested, however, that some competence decisions could be made simultaneously with commitment decisions, thus avoiding the need for excessive recourse to the courts. It also ruled that a guardian should be appointed for an incompetent refusing patient, and that the guardian is authorized to decide whether or not the patient should accept medications, using the celebrated Massachusetts "substituted consent" approach.

Thus, there are now at least two substantially different lines of cases, one severely limiting the right to refuse and relying heavily on *Romeo*, the other assuring a modestly limited right to refuse.

Conclusion

What then is the present effect of law on the administration of antipsychotic medications for involuntarily hospitalized mental patients?

In the early 1970s two federal lower courts, followed by several other federal and state courts, boldly declared a constitutional right to refuse, qualified by reasonably rigorous and necessary exceptions. Higher courts, while acknowledging the right, restricted it in such a way as to give hospitals greater flexibility to medicate, a flexibility denied in the lower courts for fear of abuse.

Then the U.S. Supreme Court not only refused to declare the constitutional right but announced a doctrine of deference to professional judgment, which could be, and was, used to transform the right to refuse into a mere right to object. Thus, emphasis was shifted from refusal to quality of care, but without judicial guidelines defining acceptable quality. Some federal courts have already deferred to the states to define quality of care for themselves, thus withdrawing almost entirely from the scene. Other federal courts may yet respond to efforts to have them define quality of care in federal constitutional terms.

In the state courts, particularly in Massachusetts, the legal doctrine of refusal persists. These state-announced rights may rest upon state common law or on statutory or constitutional doctrine. To the extent that they are not based on the federal constitution, their validity is independent of federal constitutional law, although state courts and legislatures are notoriously influenced by the U.S. Supreme Court's decisions. To the extent that state decisions rely on federal doctrine, they may have become anachronistic and subject to change. The evolution of state doctrine should be watched with great interest.

All of this is doctrine. But doctrine does not automatically translate into practice. What has been the practical consequence of this patchwork quilt of doctrine?

There is little empirical data on the outcome of right to refuse cases. Available data from New Jersey, Massachusetts, and elsewhere indicate that refusals are relatively few, and even fewer are successful. Thus, apart from doctrine, the right to refuse does not seem to have been honored as patients' lawyers intended, anticipated, and hoped. Thus, it is probably fair to regard the right to refuse as a legal chimera, a right that exists, if at all, on paper but not in actual practice.

Why has the right to refuse not flourished? In the absence of empirical data, but on the basis of informal information, one can speculate that stiff resistance from hospital doctors and staff has made the path so difficult as to discourage all but the hardiest —and perhaps most ill—refuser. Ironically, the exceptional persistence of hard-core refusers tends to be perceived as confirming their irrationality and thus to support a basic argument of those who oppose the right to refuse.

Mental patients are a particularly vulnerable and helpless group of resisters. Many do not dare or wish to refuse in the first place. Others are persuaded or coerced to withdraw refusals. The right to refuse places a premium on persistent, vigorous, and rational refusing. It seems to be a misplaced emphasis.

Is all lost, then? Have the cases accomplished only a legal mirage, a right but not an effective remedy? The answer to this question is not yet clear, if it ever will be.

Reliable, trustworthy, and unbiased observers say that the assertion of the much-publicized and dramatized right to refuse has, in effect, performed a powerful heuristic function in alerting, sensitizing, and even frightening doctors and hospital administrators into an awareness of the poor quality of medication administration and the necessity to significantly improve the quality of medical care. Thus, in hospitals throughout the country, including those in states that have had no medication litigation, the administration of medication has improved. No one has, as yet, defined or measured the extent of improvement, nor is it certain that states will not backslide once legal pressure is removed.

It appears, therefore, that while the courts have not fulfilled the precise task originally demanded of them, they have established a different form of right and have participated in an effective public morality play in which system shortcomings have been dramatized and a way to improve has been shown. Right to refuse litigation may therefore have been moderately successful, but in an unanticipated way.

References

Appelbaum, P. & Gutheil, T. (1979), Rotting with their rights on: Constitutional theory and clinical reality in drug refusal by psychiatric patients. *Bull. Am. Acad. Psychiatry Law* 7: 308–315.

Brooks, A. (1980), The constitutional right to refuse antipsychotic medications. *Bull. Am. Acad. Psychiatry Law* 8: 179–221.

Davis v. Hubbard (1980), 506 F.Supp. 915 (N.D. Ohio).

Diamond, R. (1985), Drugs and the quality of life: The patient's point of view. *J. Clin. Psychiatry* 46: 29–35.

Doudera, A. & Swazey, J., eds. (1982), *Refusing Treatment in Mental Health Institutions—Values in Conflict*. Ann Arbor, Mich.: AUPHA Press.

Estroff, S. (1981), *Making It Crazy: An Ethnography of Psychiatric Clients in an American Community*. Berkeley: University of California Press.

Gelman, S. (1983–1984), Mental hospital drugging—Atomistic and structural remedies. *Cleveland State Law Rev.* 32: 221–261.

———— (1984), Mental hospital drugs, professionalism, and the constitution. *Georgetown Law J.* 72: 1725–1784.

Gutheil, T. (1985), *Rogers v. Commissioner:* Do multiple "wrongs" make patients' rights? In: *Legal Encroachment on Psychiatric Practice*, ed. S. Rachlin, pp. 35–45. San Francisco: Jossey Bass.

Halleck, S. (1978), *The Treatment of Emotional Disorders*. New York: Jason Aronson.

In re B (1977), 156 N.J. Super. 231, 383 A.2d 760.

Klerman G. (1979), National trends in hospitalization. *Hosp. Community Psychiatry* 30: 110–114.

Lipton, A. & Simon, F. (1985), Psychiatric diagnosis in a state hospital: Manhattan State revisited. *Hosp. Community Psychiatry* 36: 368–373.

Mills v. Rogers (1982), 457 U.S. 291.

New Jersey Dept. of the Public Advocate, Div. of Mental Health Advocacy (1982), Amicus curiae brief in *Mills v. Rogers*, 102 S. Ct. 2442.

———— (1983), Notice of motion for further proceedings on remand in *Rennie v. Klein*, civil action No. 77-2624, U.S. District Court, District of New Jersey, December 21.

Ozarin, L. et al. (1976), A quarter century of psychiatric care: 1950–1974: A statistical review. *Hosp. Community Psychiatry* 27: 515–516.

Project Release v. Prevost (1983), 722 F.2d 960 (2d Cir.).

R.A.J. v. Miller (1984), 590 F.Supp. 1319 (N.D. Texas).

Rennie v. Klein (1978), 462 F.Supp. 1131 (D.N.J.).

———— (1979), 476 F.Supp. 1294 (D.N.J.).

———— (1981), 653 F.2d 836 (3d Cir.) (en banc).

———— (1982), 458 U.S. 1119.

———— (1983), 720 F.2d 266 (3d Cir.) (en banc).

Rogers v. Okin (1979), 478 F.Supp. 1342 (D. Mass.).

———— (1980), 634 F.2d 650 (1st Cir.).

Rogers v. Commissioner of Mental Health (1983), 390 Mass. 489, 458 N.E. 2d 308.

Slovenko, R. On legal aspects of tardive dyskinesia. *J. Psychiatry Law* 7: 295–330.

Stensvad v. Reivitz (1985), F.Supp. (D. Wis.).

Youngberg v. Romeo (1982), 457 U.S. 307, 102 S. Ct. 2452, 73 L. Ed. 2d 28.

Zander, T. (1977), Prolixin Decanoate: Big brother by injection? *J. Psychiatry Law* 5: 55–75.

Notes on Contributors

LAURENCE TANCREDI, Kraft Eidman Professor of Medicine and the Law and Director of the Health Law Program at the University of Texas Health Science Center at Houston, is Editor of *Ethical Issues in Epidemiologic Research*, volume 7 of *Series in Psychosocial Epidemiology*. Dr. Tancredi has written numerous books and papers on ethics, law, and psychiatry. He received his medical degree from the University of Pennsylvania School of Medicine and his law degree from Yale. From 1972–74, he was Senior Professional Associate at the Institute of Medicine of the National Academy of Sciences and served from 1979–81 as Chairman of the Council on Governmental Policy and the Law of the American Psychiatric Association. He has served on the Steering Committee on Medical Injury Compensation of the National Academy of Sciences, was a member of the National Council for Health Care of the Department of Health and Human Services, and was a consultant to the American Bar Association's Commission on Medical Professional Liability. He was co-chairperson of the Medical-Legal Research Committee of the Department of Health, Education and Welfare and is currently on the Editorial Advisory Board, Annual Bibliography of Bioethics, Kennedy Institute of Bioethics. Dr. Tancredi's current address is: The University of Texas Health Science Center at Houston, Health Law Program, 1200 Herman Pressler Drive, Suite 901, Houston, TX 77030.

NATALIE ABRAMS was formerly Assistant Professor of Philosophy in the Philosophy and Medicine Program at New York University Medical Center and then Law Clerk for the U.S. Court of Appeals, 2d Circuit, Chambers of Judge Lawrence W. Pierce. She is now an associate at the law firm of Paul, Weiss, Rifkind, Wharton, and Garrison, 345 Park Avenue, New York, NY 10154.

ALEXANDER D. BROOKS is the Justice Joseph Weintraub Professor of Law, Rutgers Law School, 15 Washington Street, Newark, NJ 07102. His major book, *Law, Psychiatry and the Men-*

tal Health System (1974 and 1980 Supplement), published by Little, Brown, received the American Psychiatric Association Guttmacher Award in 1975.

SPENCER ETH is Assistant Professor of Psychiatry at the University of California at Los Angeles, Clinical Assistant Professor of Psychiatry at the University of Southern California, and Director of Clinical Services, Mental Health Clinic, Veterans Administration Medical Center, West Los Angeles, CA 90073.

JACOB JAY LINDENTHAL is Professor and Chief of Behavioral Sciences in the Department of Psychiatry and Mental Health Sciences, University of Medicine and Dentistry, New Jersey Medical School, New Jersey Institute of Technology, 100 Bergen Street, Newark, NJ 07103.

ROBERT MICHELS is Professor and Chairman of the Department of Psychiatry, Cornell University Medical College, 525 East 68th Street, New York, NY 10021, and Psychiatrist-in-Chief of The New York Hospital.

WALTER REICH is Research Psychiatrist and Program Director of The Staff College of the National Institute of Mental Health, Lecturer in Psychiatry at Yale University, and Chairman of the Medical and Biological Sciences, Washington School of Psychiatry. His current address is: The Staff College of the National Institute of Mental Health, Room 15-81, 5600 Fishers Lane, Rockville, MD 20857.

LEE N. ROBINS is Professor of Sociology in Psychiatry in the Department of Psychiatry, Washington University School of Medicine, 4940 Audubon Avenue, St. Louis, MO 63110.

ANDREW EDMUND SLABY, an epidemiologist and psychiatrist, is Professor of Psychiatry and Human Behavior at Brown University. He has authored and co-authored numerous books, papers, and chapters on crisis-oriented therapy, characteristics of individuals in crisis, diagnostic psychiatry, emergency psychiatry, and general hospital psychiatry. Present research interests include characteristics of individual adaptation to life-threatening illness and harbingers of and modes of adaptation to adolescent suicide. Currently, he is Psychiatrist-in-Chief of the Rhode Island and Women and Infants Hospitals, Providence, RI 02902.

CLAUDEWELL S. THOMAS is Chairman, Department of Psychiatry and Human Behavior, Clarence R. Drew Post Graduate Medical School, 1720 E. 120th Street, Los Angeles, CA 90059.

DAVID N. WEISSTUB is Professor of Law, Osgoode Hall Law School of York University, Toronto, and Titulaire Professor of Psychiatry, Université de Montréal, Montreal, 10905 Est, Boulevard Henri-Bourassa, Montréal, Québec H1C 1H1.